Praise for
Mothering the Mother

"A comprehensive exploration of postpartum traditions that emphasize the importance of nurturing mothers during their most vulnerable times. From traditional recipes to rituals, this book highlights sisterhood and the need for comprehensive care that honors both the mother and the newborn."

—from the Foreword by Erykah Badu,
five-time GRAMMY Award winner,
singer/songwriter, and holistic healer

"This wonderful book is rooted in ancestral knowledge and reminds us that to 'mother the mother' is both a sacred healing practice and a radical act of reclaiming life for Black women and their families. A must-read for mothers-to-be and the women who care for them."

—Byllye Avery, founder, Black Women's
Health Imperative

"This brilliant, complete, compassionate work clearly gives Black women a blueprint for survival, thriving, and holistic joy."

—Michael W. Twitty, culinary historian, educator, and
James Beard Award–winning author of
The Cooking Gene

"*Mothering the Mother* is filled with the cultural wisdom that we so desperately lack in modern society. This book feels like heart-to-heart elder wisdom delivered at the perfect time to save lives, relationships, and tradition."

—Pānquetzani, she/her, healer, teacher, and author of *Thriving Postpartum*

"This is cultural memory made actionable; it reads like a love letter and works like a handbook. As a midwife and maternal-health advocate, I recognize a landmark text when I see one. I highly recommend this life-affirming tome to every family and every caregiver I know."

—Jennie Joseph, midwife, activist, educator, elder; founder and president of Commonsense Childbirth

"This book will *heal* not only postpartum bodies, but relationships within families, communities, and even our country hungering to feel whole once again. Mother Shafia shows us how to do this starting at the very beginning of life."

—Ananda Lowe, coauthor of *The Doula Guide to Birth*

"I learned everything I know about being a midwife from the powerful, beautiful Black midwives who took me under their wings, with Mama Shafia being the first. The wisdom you hold in your hands is timeless, woven from generations of love, faith, and practical knowledge. It will not only enrich your life now, but in ways that will unfold over years to come, in moments you cannot yet imagine."

—Aviva Romm, MD, midwife, author of *The Natural Pregnancy Book* and *Natural Health After Birth*

"In *Mothering the Mother*, Mama Shafia Monroe has woven together personal narratives, traditional practices, and recipes to support mothers. It is an important contribution that carefully documents practices that western medicine has attempted to erase."

—Monica R. McLemore, PhD, MPH,
RN, FADLN

"We do not want our mothers just to survive, we want them to thrive! Sis. Shafia Monroe brings it all home in *Mothering the Mother: African American Postpartum Traditions, Recipes, and Healing*. She brings back the sense of 'yes we can.'"

—Ayesha K. Mustafaa, managing
editor, *Muslim Journal*; instructor,
Mass Communications Department,
Tougaloo College

"Sister Shafia Monroe is an internationally acclaimed midwife not because of what she does, but how she does it. She continually reminds us that that carrying, birthing, and caring for a new soul requires that each mother receives intentional care, rituals, and food based on traditional healing beliefs and practices. *Mothering the Mother* is her gift to everyone who accepts the responsibility of being a part of this process. Thanks to this book, even though Sister Shafia cannot personally mother every mother, her presence can be felt because she is telling us exactly what she would do if she could be there . . . and what the Ancestors expect when they continue to send new life into our world. Ashe."

—Kathryn Hall-Trujillo, aka
Mama Katt, founder of Birthing
Project USA

"Each page of *Mothering the Mother* is word medicine. Wisdom, practical recipes, talk-story, well-researched facts, prayers, and a deep dive into African American culture, written in such a way that I felt wrapped in a warm soft blanket of love. Postpartum is a sacred opportunity for healing individual women, families, and communities. Mama Shafia has offered up her book, which I believe will help revive the culture of African American postpartum traditions for generations to come, while saving MotherBaby's lives."

—Ibu Robin, midwife, founder of
Bumi Sehat Foundation, 2011 CNN
"Hero of the Year," and Ashoka Fellow

"*Mothering The Mother* is a timely, extensively researched, and easy-to-read book that succeeds in thoroughly documenting and honoring the practices, traditions, and ancestral wisdom of historic Black midwives in the American South, for improving the postpartum experience."

—Linda Janet Holmes, coauthor of
*Listen to Me Good: The Story of an
Alabama Midwife*

"Mama Shafia, as she is lovingly known, has written this book with so much tenderness and care for us! May women everywhere be valued and nurtured in the way Shafia has shown us, and may we thrive joyfully as we journey through the birthing process and motherhood!"
—Dr. Jewel L. Crawford

Mothering
the Mother

Mothering the Mother

African American Postpartum
Traditions, Recipes, and Healing

Shafia Monroe

balance

New York   Boston

Balance
Hachette Book Group
1290 Avenue of the Americas
New York, NY 10104
GCP-Balance.com
@GCPBalance

First Edition: January 2026

Balance is an imprint of Grand Central Publishing. The Balance name and logo are registered trademarks of Hachette Book Group, Inc.

The publisher is not responsible for websites (or their content) that are not owned by the publisher.

The Hachette Speakers Bureau provides a wide range of authors for speaking events. To find out more, go to hachettespeakersbureau.com or email HachetteSpeakers@hbgusa.com.

Balance books may be purchased in bulk for business, educational, or promotional use. For information, please contact your local bookseller or the Hachette Book Group Special Markets Department at special.markets@hbgusa.com.

Postpartum Recuperation illustration © 2014 Shafia Monroe Consulting. www.ShafiaMonroe.com.
Print book interior design by Sheryl Kober.

Library of Congress Control Number: 2025039010

ISBNs: 978-0-306-83543-8 (trade paperback), 978-0-306-83544-5 (ebook)

Printed in the United States of America

LSC-C

Printing 1, 2025

To my mother, Yvonne Delilia Kenion Monroe, who loved
to read, visit the library, and read me bedtime stories. She
modeled for me the power of the written word and taught that
important things are written down and kept safe in books.

Contents

A LOVE LETTER TO BLACK MOTHERS

Dear Mother,

Let me be the first to tell you that you are beautiful, blessed, and loved. Motherhood is a cherished gift, and you deserve to be honored, protected, cared for, consoled, and uplifted by society. I want to help you rejoice in motherhood, heal after childbirth, and bond with your new baby.

In African culture, motherhood is the epitome of sacredness and power. Therefore, you are sacred, and you are powerful. I see you, and I am familiar with the journey of motherhood that you will travel for the rest of your life. You made a sacrifice to bring your baby into the world as a gift, and you deserve all the love and support that comes with being a mother. You deserve to receive the help you need to raise your baby and regain your strength after childbirth. I know and believe the African proverb "It takes a village to raise a child" is true. I know all too well, having raised seven children, that motherhood is a village effort. This support held me up when I least expected it but needed it most, so please accept the help from your village for you and your baby's sake.

If you were my daughter, I would be there to help you and the father of your child during your birth; I would be so excited and proud of you. And I would remind you of our rich tradition of birthing without fear and believing in our bodies to do everything perfectly. And I would say the prayer of thanksgiving to bless you while you held and nursed your baby for the first time.

While in the bed, I would hand-feed you my special postpartum coconut curry chicken soup that I made to warm your insides, give you energy, and begin your postpartum recovery to wellness. I would practice African American postpartum care to keep you happy, prevent postpartum depression, and help you produce abundant breastmilk. I would apply the African American belly wrap to hold your uterus in place while it shrinks to its pre-pregnancy size and back down into your pelvis.

I would wait on you hand and foot because I love you so much. I would care for you so you can love, smell, kiss, nurse, and marvel at your new baby. I would be there to answer any of your baby care questions, let you rest while I bathe and change the baby, and I would teach you how to safely co-sleep, like I did with you and your siblings, for infant health, easy nursing, and optimal rest.

After you complete the forty-two-day lying-in period, we would honor you and this milestone with a beautiful naming ceremony. This ceremony is an ancient African ritual, similar to a Christian Baptism or Islamic Aqiqah, where we introduce the baby to the larger community, hold a dinner for family and neighbors to show gratitude to the Creator for a healthy mother and baby, and ask for the attendees' blessings for the newborn. Extended family and close friends would come to meet the baby and bring gifts for them as well as money for you. We would dress you up like a queen in new clothes, smoked with hints of rose, frankincense, and myrrh. You would feel happy and content. Because I mothered you for forty-two days and fed you nutrient-rich postpartum soups, gave you regular massages, sat you in herbal postpartum baths, allowed you to sleep well, and loved and served you consistently, you would be a bright, shining, rested, happy, strong, and glowing new mother, ready to receive your guests. And still, you would be served during the naming *ceremony; all you would need to do is sit, eat, and show off your baby—and even then, someone else could do that for you if you chose.*

But since I can't be there with you, I humbly offer you this book. Its purpose is to show you the ancestral ways of loving, healing, and caring for yourself and blessing you and your baby during your postpartum period. It grows out of the wisdom and creativity of our people. I am so blessed to be able to play a role in helping you get what you deserve: time to rest, heal, and enjoy your baby.

Congratulations, dear one, and God bless you, your baby, and your entire family.

I love you,
Mama Shafia

The elders say that what you go through in life can mold you for the better. I say to you, own your greatness as a mother. I will share with you the mantra I wrote for myself years ago to remember that my life, with all its emotions and challenges, is amazing: "I am divinely guided, I am truly blessed, and I am living my success right now." I invite you to say this mantra throughout the day. Remember that you are divinely guided in all things. It all works out. You are blessed.

Foreword

Peace and well wishes to all.

    It is with great honor that I introduce *Mothering the Mother*, a vital resource that explores the sacred traditions, recipes, and holistic healing practices that have carried and long supported African American mothers during the postpartum period.

    I am a birth and end-of-life doula, and none of this would have been possible without the profound teachings of Mother Shafia Monroe, whose teachings are invaluable and whose heart is light. My journey to this moment has been deeply influenced by all the strong women who raised me.

    As the tenth born and first daughter in my family, I carry the legacy of those who came before me with purpose. This maternal lineage is not just a familial connection; it is a scientific bond rooted in the very fabric of our being—the mitochondrial DNA shared among women, linking us to our ancestors and grounding us in the richness of our magical heritage.

    In *Mothering the Mother*, Mother Shafia presents a comprehensive exploration of postpartum traditions that emphasize the importance of nurturing mothers during their most vulnerable times. The practices outlined within are steeped in cultural significance, serving to strengthen not only physical recovery but also emotional and spiritual well-being. From traditional recipes to rituals that promote healing, this book highlights sisterhood and the need for comprehensive care that honors both the mother and the newborn.

It offers gentleness.

As you engage with this text, you will discover methods that have sustained families and communities for generations.

Our tribe-based traditions are important and relevant; they continue to resonate. Mother Shafia's insights offer a framework for understanding the complexities of postpartum care in the African American community, reminding us that to support a mother is to support the entire family unit. This book is a crucial exploration of the intersection of culture, health, and maternal care. Mother Shafia invites us to reflect on the practices that have nourished and empowered all women throughout time. This book is special. Thank you, Mother Shafia.

I am so honored to be among what I call the Welcoming Committee. Welcome to motherhood, welcome to *Mothering the Mother*.

Peace peace,
Erykah Badu

Introduction

HOW I BECAME "QUEEN MOTHER" OF A MIDWIFE MOVEMENT

EVEN THOUGH BOTH MY PARENTS ARE AFRICAN AMERICANS, I LOVE to tell people that I am bicultural because my mother was a second-generation Bostonian Catholic. My father was a rural, foot-washing Alabamian Baptist. I lived in a dual world, and I benefited from both cultures. This duality, as well as the proud claiming of my African heritage, was the foundation from which I was anointed as a healer, environmentalist, and midwife.

With Daddy being from the South, he wanted to eat grits every morning, and Mama, a Northern Catholic, wanted fish on Friday and was fine eating oatmeal, Cream of Wheat, or cold cereal for breakfast. My father taught my siblings and me the proper call-and-response to show respect to our parents and elders. When he called out to one of us, our expected response was either, "Yes, sir" or "Yes, sir, I will be right there." Meanwhile, my mother supported me in going outside the lines of what was expected of a Black woman. She instilled in me the importance of asking questions, always reading the fine print before signing any document, and, of course, the value of helping people and giving back to our community.

Reflecting back, I can see that my dad had particular conservative traditions that reflect family values and daily structure while at the other end of the spectrum, my mother was a liberal who believed in bodily autonomy and equal rights for women. I see now how this all ties into African American postpartum traditions, which have a lot of structure and respect for family roles while also celebrating and supporting Black women's bodies, autonomy, and wellness.

I learned the African tradition of eating hot meals from my dad, while I first learned how to care for newborns by watching my mother. After bathing my baby niece, who was about eight weeks old, my mother would place her on a thick, dry towel on our dining room table and massage her entire body with warmed oil. I remember my mother stretching my niece's arms and legs while oiling her skin, rubbing her hands in a circle around her little head, down her forehead, and around to the back of her head for at least five minutes. When I asked my mother what she was doing, she told me that you must shape the head to make it round. At the end of the massage, my mother would hold my niece upside down by her legs. She told me you must stretch the baby out so they will be strong-legged with good posture. During the entire ritual, my niece never cried. Decades later, when I made a visit to a village in Senegal, West Africa, I saw a mother massaging and stretching her baby in a similar way.

I had simple traditions growing up. Before I walked out the front door for school each morning, I had to read out loud, to my mother, a note that she had taped to the door. She titled it "Don't forget the three magic words," and it read, "Please, thank you, and I am sorry." At the end of the list, it said, "I love you." I went to school with that message five days a week—please, thank you, I am sorry, and I love you. These words have been instrumental in my successfully navigating the world.

It was important to my father that my siblings and I spent time with our grandmother and learned the rural Southern culture, so every summer, he drove us from Boston to Alabama. While there, my father showed me how to respect the land by making fires in certain places and putting them out properly, how to make a bow and arrow, how to cut and smoke the pine tree branches to keep the mosquitoes away, and how to breathe in the pine smoke for healthy lungs. He had my cousin teach me how to saddle and ride horses, and even how to ride bareback. He taught me not to be afraid to ride through the woods, how to avoid water moccasins when swimming in the creek, how to shoot a shotgun, how to bring the cows in at night, and how to fish. He even taught me about waiting until the full moon to plant crops and cut your hair.

I learned about African American healing recipes and postpartum traditions because my parents and extended family recognized the healer in me, and they taught me that healing was part of my legacy as an African American. As a child, I could feel uneasiness in people and animals, and I gravitated toward those who I felt needed my help. I remember the shy new girl who arrived in my first-grade class with a heavy smell that came from her parents putting Sulfur8 in her hair to make it grow. The other students teased and ostracized her because they said she smelled funny. I knew this was cruel and wrong, so I played with her during recess, walked with her after school, and let her know that I would be her friend. My propensity to help others was the catalyst that led me to midwifery at age sixteen and catching babies solo by age twenty-four. I wanted to help families experience positive and loving births.

The time period I was born in also had a hand in shaping the person I ended up becoming. I was born during the Civil Rights Movement, the rise of the Black Panther Party, and the popularization of the Nation of Islam—the period known as the Black Power

Movement. This taught me about the injustices afflicted upon Black people, including the Tuskegee experiment, Black maternal and infant mortality, and the illegal hysterectomies that were performed to sterilize Black women.

The Civil Rights and Black Power Movements affirmed what my parents had taught me: I am important, I matter, I am beautiful, my opinion counts, I should be proud of my African heritage, and I am a leader. It revived a consciousness in many Black people to turn to our culture for solutions, education, spirituality, and health. During this time, I became interested in Black Southern healing traditions. I wanted to reclaim what was taken from us because of the Transatlantic Slave Trade. The enslavement of African people destroyed our languages, family structure, religions, healthy traditional diets, birth and postpartum traditions, and parenting practices. I was called to learn Black postpartum traditions to empower my community and find solutions to the historical trauma of Black infant and maternal mortality rates, and in 1973, I began looking for information on traditional African and African American birth culture, creating a paradigm shift in public health and, more importantly, in the Black community.

As I studied Black birth and postpartum traditions, I learned that African mothers have a sophisticated method of massaging and stretching the baby's body, molding their head, and shaping their face and buttocks for proper alignment and development. This immediately brought me back to my mother massaging my newborn niece. Baby massages and head shaping were common among Black Americans because it was passed down from our enslaved African ancestors, who taught this ritual as an act of love and infant development. My grandmother, and all the women and men of my Southern family, had similar traditions to those of the twentieth-century Black midwifery practices: She was clean, spiritual, religious, disciplined, dependable, and respected, and she was the go-to person for guidance on how to build a healthy family. Black midwives of the twentieth century held a status comparable to that of a preacher, and some say her status superseded the preacher's, with stories of a pastor giving up his seat to the midwife when she arrived at a dinner table. This is a testimony to her status within her community. After all, the midwife most likely delivered that very preacher. The community respected her as their link and upholder of ancient birthing practices, with preconception and postnatal rituals taught to her from previous generations of African midwives, herbalists, and healers.

My paternal grandmother was born May 15, 1891, in Pollard, Alabama. As I learned more about African healing, I observed that my grandmother practiced a lot of the same traditions, knowing or unknowingly. She lived by the cosmos and nature. She used water as medicine, particularly for drinking, cleaning, and bathing. She was meticulous, grooming me in her traditional way that focused on hygiene, spirituality, diet, relationships, and work—like how women lived in Africa. Her day began at early dawn, and she was often well into her schedule by sunrise, including having dinner cooking on the stove. She taught me to cook early before the sun hits the highest point in the sky because she said it was too hot to be in the kitchen then. She said dinner should be ready to eat before the sun sets, that it was better for your health and helped you avoid digestion problems. Though she worked hard, she always stopped at noon, or the hottest time of day, to rest. She would sit on the porch with water and relax for one to two hours. As she got older, she would lay in her bed and take a nap.

Like my grandmother and many of our African female ancestors, Black women carried themselves through the matriarchal linkage. They were businesswomen, healers, midwives, and landowners.

They made and controlled their own wealth. They bought land and passed inheritances through their line. My grandmother birthed at home, buried an infant, and practiced all of the traditional African American postpartum traditions and rituals, like not sitting on cold steps or chairs, eating greens and protein soups, drinking sassafras tea, using turpentine and spider webs for healing, sewing menstrual pads, and using a belly wrap during her postpartum time.

I could see that all these traditions had not been lost in her time, and they are now more important than ever to help Black mothers have the most healing postpartum period possible and to help their families know how to care for them and the new baby.

Today, over 1,200 women die every year due to pregnancy or childbirth-related causes, and approximately 60,000 women face severe, life-threatening complications.[1] Thousands more suffer postpartum conditions that negatively impact their quality of life, such as chronic backaches, headaches, fatigue, perineal or pelvic pain, mastitis, cracked nipples, hemorrhoids, prolapsed uterus, hemorrhage, depression, infection, uterine inversion, constipation, painful healing of an episiotomy, pain or infection from a cesarean section, bladder infection, urinary incontinence, postpartum-induced hypertension (PIH), and iron-deficient anemia. Without treatment, these conditions can worsen and affect the long-term health of a new mother. Postpartum illness disproportionately affects Black mothers, who are three times more likely to die from childbirth-related causes than their non-Hispanic, white counterparts and more than twice as likely to experience severe postpartum health conditions. This health inequity exists irrespective of socioeconomic status and education level, pointing to more profound, systemic issues.[2]

Since my early days of learning to ride horses and reciting the magic words (please, thank you, and I am sorry), I have birthed seven of my own babies, caught hundreds more as a midwife, trained over five thousand doulas, spent thousands of hours counseling new parents, and devoted myself to researching the postpartum traditions that were lost—the ones that Black women and the Black community so desperately need to effectively take charge of our health within a medical system that disregards the importance of family and tradition in postpartum healing. We need to give Black mothers the legacy of beauty, confidence, health, and faith in our bodies and our ability to fully recover from birth.

Mothering the Mother is built on the rich history of our African American postpartum traditions. It revives best practices, community responsibility, and African American foodways for proper healing and is a direct link to our African ancestry. It connects African American mothers to our culture, reduces isolation, and teaches what foods to eat, how to be grateful, how to have faith in God for our ability to mother and heal at the same time, and how to use rest as a form of worship. Above all, it teaches that having our baby next to us and on us is a natural form of healing.

Reclaiming our postpartum traditions is critical in an environment that devalues Black motherhood and, historically, gave Black enslaved women less than twenty-four hours post-birth to return to the field or the "big house." When the African American midwife was eradicated from her community in the 1920s, it created a legacy of birth injustices, as our healing practices, mothering traditions, and beautification rituals were lost.

Honoring the sacredness of motherhood is the core of this book for two reasons: (1) To affirm that the love and respect of the mother is the foundation of African/Black culture, for a healthy self and society; and (2) to acknowledge the historical trauma that Black mothers have endured on US soil, which began with our babies being sold from us while they were nursing at our breasts and continues with the racial profiling of our children today. The subconscious hypervigilance to protect our children can keep us in a fight-flight-or-freeze state. This negatively impacts the postpartum experience because chronic stress impairs hormonal balance and weakens the immune system. Implementing African American postpartum traditions, foods, and healing can help regulate hormones, reduce stress, and create a state of whole-body well-being.

In Part 1, I introduce the Granny Midwife and the rich history and traditions she kept alive through Sankofa, the West African concept that tells us to look to the past to inform the future. In Part 2, I share details about several traditions for postpartum healing, such as resting, staying hydrated, applying heat to the body, and using herbs for holistic rejuvenation. And in Part 3, I give you healthy traditional recipes and rituals you can use and adapt with your family to aid in easeful postpartum healing. This is Sankofa in real time, and it is my hope that it will help you feel loved, honored, and blessed throughout your postpartum recuperation.

THE PRAYER OF THE
MISSISSIPPI
Black Midwives

Our forebearers spent their lives praying for a good life for our future generations. The Mississippi Black midwives were known to pray, "Our heavenly father, the author and finisher of our lives, we give thee thanks for health and strength and all the joys of life. We pray that thou would bless the mothers and fathers everywhere." We stand on the shoulders of those who came before us. Honoring our past and practicing ancestral traditions is one way to honor their work on our behalf and benefit from their lessons learned.

PART ONE

Thanking Our Ancestors: The Roots of African American Postpartum Care

CHAPTER 1

Reviving the Lost Traditions of the African American Granny Midwife

*Transitioning to motherhood is natural and beautiful. We honor
the Granny Midwives who came before us and offered wisdom
and support. We thank the Granny Midwives who taught us how
to relax, not be afraid, and ask for help so we can enjoy our babies
and our new position as mothers.*

*You deserve to know and be proud of our postpartum legacy
of love, healing, and ritual-based medicine that was taught to us
by the Granny Midwife, which was passed on to her by our African ancestors so you can be well, happy, and confident mothering
your newborn.*

BEFORE I BECAME A MIDWIFE, I WAS DETERMINED TO BECOME AN
obstetrician until, one day, my uncle Mel asked me, "What about
becoming a midwife?" I had never heard that word before, so I told
him I would go to the library and look it up. The librarian gave me
a bunch of books. Sitting at a big table, I came across the phrase
"Granny Midwife" and its definition: a well-respected elder Black
woman in the rural South who believed God called her to provide
childbirth services based on ancestral practices. I was moved when

I read about how Granny Midwives never turned anyone away and how the community looked up to them. It all resonated with my soul, and I was hooked. I could feel a spiritual bridge open, connecting me, my past, and my future with midwifery and spiritual healing. I knew I had to become a midwife and practice like the Granny Midwives did to honor them and bring healing to my community.

However, after completing my midwifery training, I quickly discovered that very few in my field spoke of Granny Midwives or Black birthing and postpartum traditions. I don't think they knew this information existed. I was committed to learning more about our cultural ways of taking care of a mother and her newborn after birth, so in my early years of practice, I traveled often to attend postpartum workshops, hoping to learn rituals and practices that felt relevant and familiar to me and the mothers in my community. I'd sit in rooms full of white women, with minimal women of color, and listen to in-depth descriptions of postpartum philosophies and practices from other cultures. In the early years, Mexican postpartum traditions were very prominent in the midwifery community, with teachings on soups, rebozo rituals to close the bones, and body wrapping. Then Chinese medicine, with acupuncture, placental medicine, and Mother Roasting, seemed to take center stage. Over the years, I learned about the Japanese Ansei tradition of staying with the mother after birth, the Swedish postpartum visiting nurse, and the East Indian postpartum massage. At the end of each workshop, I would go home to my predominantly Black community to care for Black mothers and their newborns, with the longing to offer them postpartum traditions that were culturally relevant to them and spiritually connected to our ancestors.

It was as if we did not have a postpartum culture when history shows that we did—and still do. In fact, up until the 1950s, African American postpartum traditions were the dominant type of care in the Southern United States for both Black and white mothers. If you were pregnant or postpartum in the Southern United States in the twentieth century, you and your baby were most likely cared for by a Black midwife, who leaned on traditions and rituals stemming from the diverse cultures of the African continent.

Granny Midwives, as they were known, were well-respected elder women who provided compassionate care to help women birth their babies with dignity. After birth, they supported the new mother deeper than a modern-day postpartum doula would, by providing ancient practices to honor motherhood, compassionately care for babies, and keep mother and baby clean, nourished, and well-fed with baths, massages, and appropriate herbs to help them heal physically and mentally from the effects of birth. The Granny Midwife was a fusion of African healing, spirituality, practical instinct, and intuition.

Her midwifery practices were standard until the early twentieth century, when they were abandoned and replaced by Western medical standards due to an explicit campaign to delegitimize and stigmatize Black Granny Midwives. The seed of doubt was purposefully planted by those in the emerging white medical system, who passed judgment on Black postpartum traditions. This campaign to vilify the Granny Midwife was led by public health and medical professionals who told Black women that their customs had no scientific value, accused them of practicing superstition, or cajoled them by saying, "Why do you want to practice those old granny backward ways? You're too smart for that." Over time, with the subtle and overt pressure to conform to the white medicalization of birth and their definition of postpartum care, we began doubting our ancestral ways, eventually losing touch with much of the knowledge of our postpartum traditions and rituals and assimilating to the dominant culture of postpartum care.

Although I rarely heard mention of them at midwifery workshops, I've spent the last twenty years studying the life of the Granny Midwife and Black postpartum traditions through books, travel, documentaries, hundreds of personal interviews and oral histories, and a wealth of experience from practicing African American postpartum care on Black mothers and seeing how they recovered. Mothers who I have helped testify to how much better and stronger they feel because of African American postpartum practices.

I like to share the history of the Black Granny Midwife with every mother in my care. I share this with you now because it is part of your legacy too. The Granny Midwife's wisdom, faith, warmth, practices, prayers, and ceremonies—her connection to our history—are sacred to you, your baby, your community, and your beautiful transformation into motherhood. Different life circumstances can impact how motherhood unfolds for each of us each time we become a mother, yet there is no wrong way. What is universal in our postpartum traditions is that you deserve to be honored, loved, and helped, and it is the responsibility of the family and community to care for you.

Walking in the Footsteps of the Granny Midwife

I was once asked to be a midwife for a woman who was having her fifth baby and first home birth. On the day she gave birth, she called me once she was in active labor, and I arrived in enough time to put the collard green coconut curry chicken soup on the stove. In addition to curry powder, I added garlic, cayenne, and a salt mix for an extra postpartum benefit. In a stainless-steel pot, I simmered ginger root, comfrey, nettle leaves, and a few leaves of green sage. She had chosen to give birth in a squatting position on a quilt on the floor. Once the baby was born, she sat back in a reclining position with pillows supporting her back and began to nurse her newborn with the placenta still attached inside her uterus. As soon as she was comfortably positioned, her doula began feeding her spoonfuls of the warmed soup. She said, "Oh my God, this is delicious."

While we were waiting for the placenta to expel and as she fed the mother, my assistant midwife applied warm cloths soaked in my hot comfrey brew to the mother's vulva to provide relief, kick-start the circulation of oxygenated blood, and create immediate healing. We use comfrey, a proven postpartum herb, to heal bruised and scratched skin from birth.

The mother told me days later that she had felt so strong. She said she could literally feel strength entering her body after eating each spoonful of the soup. On my next postpartum visit, she said, "This is my fifth baby, and I never felt so good so soon after having a baby."

I gave her the traditional forty-two days of African American postpartum care. Every day, I spent three to five hours with her and her family so she could be nourished, massaged, beautified, and given time to sleep. I kept reminding her to stay in bed to prevent excess bleeding, exhaustion, and long-term body aches, and I did the chores and tasks that would allow her to stay there. I made sure she had soup, tea, water, seasonal fruit, fat, and proteins daily. I would draw her a postpartum bath, change her bedding, give her a clean gown to put on, and massage her after every bath. I would also hold the baby if he was fussy after breastfeeding so she could get at least one full hour of sleep.

Walking in the footsteps of the Granny Midwife, I remember how hard they worked to ensure the new mother returned to wellness mentally, spiritually, and physically, and that the baby was kept clean, warm, loved, and in low light for full eye development. As a modern-day Granny Midwife, my goal is to make sure the mothers in my care reach a state of complete wellness.

"Keep resting," I tell my mamas, "because that is what our culture says to do."

THE ORIGINS OF THE GRANNY MIDWIFE[1]

Starting in 1619, millions of kidnapped Africans survived the Transatlantic Slave Trade and were introduced to horrendous conditions of enslavement in the United States. Over time, the women began working to aid the sick and dying and serve birthing and postpartum women under dire conditions. They used traditional African healing practices and, when the resources they were familiar with weren't available, they were creative and inventive, using the herbs and foods they could find. This is the emergence of the African American Granny Midwife.

The African American definition of midwife originates in African languages. It is expansive in its meaning, going beyond the Eurocentric definition of "with wife" or, as often translated, "with woman." The underlying foundation of the word "midwife" in Black American culture included community healers because in African culture, the collective, not just the individual, is spiritually healed with these practices. Because Granny Midwives cared for mothers and babies as well as the sick and the dying, and more generally as a nurse to the community, she had an integrated approach to the way she provided postpartum care. These traditions of comprehensive care are supported by literature that speaks to how the postpartum period impacts everyone—mother, baby, father, children, and the entire family.

Having roots in African healing, the postpartum period was multidimensional. This intense time of postpartum traditions and rituals by the Granny Midwife signified to the community that the new mother was still at the doorway of life and death, and it was critical that she be prayed for and prayed over during the forty-two-day laying-in period. Our traditions took note of the spiritual and physical to allow the mother to come safely and fully back from the birth experience. Her care also included the newborn's emotional and spiritual safety, as well as that of the entire family.

The assault on Black motherhood has been an unfair burden, and Granny Midwives knew that our postpartum traditions and rituals could override some of the adverse outcomes. She reassured us, even in the fear of losing our children, that God was on our side and that our babies were covered in protection. She reminded us to keep our faith, to believe in good, to breathe, relax, rest, and to love and be loved. She taught us to smell our babies for emotional support, nurse our babies as much as possible, perform the naming ceremonies with prayer, and raise our children as God-conscious people as our ancestors did. We'll dive deep into the postpartum practices and techniques of Black postpartum care in Part 2, but for now, I want to share some of the key aspects of Granny Midwifery, including "Motherwit," "waiting on," the Community Mothering Model, and herbs and nourishing meals to help guide and orient your own postpartum care.

Motherwit

Being in an unfamiliar environment, the first few generations of Granny Midwives relied on what's known as "Motherwit" to navigate healing on North American shores.[2] Motherwit emerged from spiritual practices, as well as divine gifts or guidance, to know what was needed to heal the body, mind, and spirit using traditional medicine and foods. Granny Midwives used their ingenuity to identify and use the appropriate Native American and European herbs, along with the minimal African herbs they could access, such as black-eyed-pea leaves, castor oil, watermelon seeds, and okra leaves, to heal and soothe the body and spirit. They were so successful that many white Southerners trusted, and even preferred, Africans' medicine of herbs, massage, and heat over their white physicians' medical treatments, which consisted of bloodletting, leeching, amputations, and purging. White pregnant women would often call on Granny Midwives to help them during their births because they trusted their traditional African birthing practices.

Granny Midwives believed that to be successful in the work, you had to be divinely guided and maintain the ancient birthing practices and postnatal rituals, which had been passed down by the previous generations.[3] Many claimed to have been called to do this work in a dream or by God. They often came from a lineage of midwives, and they were known to say, "Midwifery runs in my family. My grandmother was a midwife, as was my mother." Granny Midwives were usually older women with life experience; had been married, divorced, or widowed; and had birthed, buried, and raised their own babies as well as others'. Some even claimed to have learned their healing practices directly from Africa.[4] Others said circumstances led them to midwifery; they saw the need, and there was no one else to do it.

They said, "Motherwit is the inner knowing; it is the belief that you can know how to do something by listening to your inner voice, using prayer, hearing the answer, observing, and acting on faith." Many of my midwife friends have told me they did things based on faith that they had never done, and it worked. Some called it the spiritual voice, and some explained it as God informing them of what to do. Regardless, Motherwit ensured that postpartum care was heavy on emotional support, spiritual rituals, intimacy, intuition, expectation, and community obligations. It was genuine holistic care. Motherwit meant knowing how to create an individualized care plan based on the birth and the mother's emotional needs. Whether the mother had a precipitous birth, a physically challenging birth, multiple births, an exceptionally long birth, a stillbirth, or was ill during pregnancy, the Granny Midwife would intuitively know what was needed to help this mama heal. This may have meant more herbal baths, other types of salves, additional foods and herbal formulas to facilitate healing, or more prayers, songs, touch, and talking.

The Granny Midwives would say that you've got to have common sense to be a midwife, and they would say it's not always what you see or hear, but what you feel—the deep knowing in your soul or spirit. For this reason, some people refer to Motherwit as the third eye. It is looking at a seemingly healthy mother yet feeling that things are not going to go well, or the opposite, like when people or the medical community offer dismal or poor outcomes, but mama feels in her gut that she or her baby will be fine. There have been times when I felt labor would begin on a particular day, and it did. The Granny Midwife also had an intuitive knowing during pregnancy about how a mother would recuperate during her postpartum period.

I think of Motherwit as an internal compass that we need to listen to and develop. Some years ago, I accepted the invitation to be the midwife for a pregnant woman having her fourth baby. All her previous births had been problem-free. I visited regularly, keeping to the standard prenatal schedule. Every visit, my Motherwit would go on high alert. Her vital signs were good, but I still felt uneasiness with her. Though she was excited about her pregnancy, she had some personal stress related to her job and cared for an ill family member, which required her to travel regularly. I remember sitting with her one day for a prenatal check, and as she was talking to me, a feeling came over me that she was not healthy, even though her and her baby's hearts were fine. I sent her to the hospital for bloodwork, and there, they discovered that she had developed an infection. She took the medicine needed to cure the illness and recovered well. I am grateful that my Motherwit kicked in, and that I listened to my inner voice that kept saying something was wrong.

We see the dismissal of our Motherwit in the preventable causes of Black maternal mortality, where a mother will go to the hospital because she feels something is not right, and her medical team will send her home saying there is nothing wrong with her, labeling her symptoms as "stress." The medical system uses that as an excuse to deny Black women adequate care when we know that underlying conditions often surface after birth, whether it's an infected cesarean section incision, a piece of the placenta left in the womb, elevated blood pressure, or blood clots. The mother often knows something is wrong. She may not be able to name what it is, but she knows it exists because of Motherwit. Unfortunately, the Westernized medical system calls that superstition and ignores what the mother says, denying her the necessary testing to confirm her concerns.

Black Women, Own Your Motherwit

You know if something is wrong with you or your baby; don't let anyone dismiss you. Insist that your healthcare provider runs more tests until your concerns are put to rest or get a second opinion. My Motherwit has served me well. When my baby daughter, my third birth, was maybe five months old, I noticed that she was not acting normally. I brought her to the hospital, and they did not find anything, but I knew something was wrong. I went back at least two more times, and they eventually discovered that she had pneumonia. I thank God for Motherwit.

Waiting On: "It's an Act of Love"

In an era when women were averaging sixteen to twenty-one births under the most inhumane conditions of enslavement, Jim Crow segregation, and lynching, the Granny Midwife was a beacon of light for postpartum families. No matter the number of pregnancies, the Granny Midwife and family "waited on" the mother each time, and she reminded everyone of this important tradition. Her presence represented culture, familiarity, love, and trust. Families knew that "she was going to be there for [them]."[5] She cared for new mothers with affection and attention to help ease the burden of worry, gave mothering advice, and engaged and honored the father. She validated Black mothering styles and practiced traditional beautification rituals to affirm the mother's beauty and soothe her emotions. "Waiting on" is a literal action, an act of love that's meant to serve the postpartum mother.

Ms. Gladys Milton, a Floridian midwife of the twentieth century, is a wonderful example of "waiting on" practices for postpartum mothers. Delivering well over two thousand babies—some say perhaps as many as three thousand—Ms. Milton provided postpartum services in the homes of her clients and sought aid for them through church and civic groups. She knew when the families she "waited on" needed resources, and she would bring them gifts to help them, honoring the family's dignity.[6]

Similarly, in her autobiography, midwife Onnie Lee Logan tells the story of the time a husband brought his wife to her home, seeking help. The wife had given birth, was bleeding, and had a deep vaginal tear. Ms. Lee told the husband to leave his wife with her for some days. She put the new mother to bed and immediately began waiting on her, first by washing her, then by applying postpartum herbs to her tear and wrapping her legs together to facilitate vaginal healing. She repeated this treatment daily, and when her husband came back to fetch her, the vaginal tear was well on its way to being healed.[7]

"Waiting on" is part of the sacred work of Black midwives, and as a result, everyone wanted to be waited on by the Granny Midwife because she provided loving, personalized, and spiritual care. This is the foundation of holistic postpartum wellness.

You Are Blessed

Postpartum is about surrendering to the natural order of the divine. Though babies are blessings in our culture and postpartum is normal, it is different for everyone. Postpartum can be simple and easy for some women and painful for others. The birth may not have gone according to your plan. Regardless, the Granny Midwife is there to remind you, as a new mother, that you are a blessed spiritual being, and your baby will bring you unimaginable blessings. The Granny Midwife is blessed to wait on you.

More Than a Baby Catcher: A Community Mothering Model

As a pillar in my community, I am called to do more than catch babies. I am asked to speak to teen girls who are interested in midwifery, talk with new mothers about their infants' first foods or how to increase breastmilk, be a listening ear and inspire others to be their best selves, honor the father and respect the grandmothers, and interact with the families' children. This is another part of the tradition that I uphold and carry on. Granny Midwives lived in the communities they served, and when people saw the Granny Midwife walking in the community, they would stop her on the street to greet her and get advice on a variety of problems. She was more than a baby catcher; she was a psychologist, dietician, loan officer, sex therapist, prayer warrior, marriage counselor, friend, and sometimes a relative to the families she served. She was an advisor on matters of the heart and social discourse and the go-to person for information on reproductive health, infertility, baby spacing, miscarriage, birth and postpartum care, relations, parenting advice, and community support.

As one account shares, "Granny was a midwife, nurse, problem solver, lawgiver, and feud solver, and she told you how it was going to go."[8] She was always on the job, always available to her community to help heal and maintain spiritual balance with advice, prayers, laying on of hands (healing touch), tonics, salves, suggestions for reproductive health, and midwifery services. She was a pillar in her community, and her advice was respected, even if it was not always followed. Her authoritative position meant she carried a heavy responsibility, which gave her a lot of respect from community members.

Her high status was tied to her spiritual call to midwifery and her ability to patiently work under harsh conditions without monetary compensation in most cases.[9] The Granny Midwife status was earned, and it came with the prestige from the African culture of respecting the elders, healers, and doers. The people trusted the Granny Midwife, they valued her input, and they were proud of what she represented for their community. The community knew she was a conduit of African birth practices and that she tried to do what God would have her do, not what she wanted to do. She was an example of how to act in a God-conscious way, a reminder and a director for creating a healthy family unit. The Granny Midwives were meticulous in keeping their homes clean and practiced the African way of personal hygiene, spirituality, diet, relationships, and work. They knew that part of healing was based on how your body felt and asserted that feeling clean lifted the spirits.

Like in many matriarchal African societies, the Granny Midwife followed the example of being a businesswoman. Despite the unfair treatment they often received at the hands of the white medical community, many of these women managed to earn incomes, control their money, buy land, and pass inheritances through their matriarchal lineage. It was common for Granny Midwives to turn their homes into a refuge, a safe space for prenatal and postpartum care and new mothers in need.[10] In this way, among others, they were part of a long tradition of community mothering, in which new mothers knew they could rely on seasoned mothers to mentor them.

Embrace Community Mothering

You need and deserve comprehensive care that offers equal attention to each phase of the postpartum period. Motherhood and mothering are sacred positions, and our experiences and stories count. We flourish as mothers by using the Community Mother

Model and relying on seasoned mothers to mentor us. As new mothers, we thrive on being validated that we are doing a good job, being fed, and being adorned by beautification rituals. Community Mothering helps us build confidence, which is essential for our mental, physical, and spiritual postpartum recovery.

Herbs and Nourishing Meals

During the twentieth century, everyone grew up harvesting and using herbs as medicine. Mint tea was customary to help with after-meal digestion, chamomile was used for stomach pains, rosemary helped your hair get thick, and mullein tea soothed coughs and congestion. It was expected that the Granny Midwives would be most knowledgeable about using herbs to improve women's reproductive health, heal after childbirth, and promote infant well-being. They grew up being given herbs for healing and later learned to use them in their work by watching the herbalists in their community and being taught by the elderly midwives they worked under. Common herbs for postpartum were dandelion root, borage, mints, lemon balm, nutmeg, and cinnamon.

A midwife was expected to have a garden with flowers, herbs, vegetables, and some chickens. Midwives kept gardens because it was the tradition, and they knew food was medicine. They wanted to help families as needed and were known to bring greens, veggies, and eggs to needy families. They would also welcome people into their gardens to grab fresh veggies. Some midwives would cook meals on Sunday and bring them to church to share with others.

Midwives would give mothers borage tea and rice porridge to help increase breastmilk supply, make the milk richer, and induce sleep. It was common for a postpartum home to smell warm as families were instructed to boil fruit, such as lemons and oranges, for the mother to drink. This was intended to help her sweat out excess water from the body and aid in her recovery from childbirth. To honor Granny Midwives, I grow many traditional herbs in my yard, like peppermint and mint because I've found that a warm cup of mint and lemon balm tea can do wonders to help a postpartum mama feel relaxed and sleepy when she's restless.

What couldn't be sourced from the midwives' gardens could usually be sourced from the nearby woods. They often used fresh herbs but would also keep the essential herbs ready by drying them or making them into tonics. When I do my doula training, I keep fresh and dried herbs on the premises for demonstration purposes, and it is always powerful when a trainee gets a headache, digestion issues, or even period cramps and I get to use herbs in real time to demonstrate how they relieve symptoms, often within hours. In one training session, a participant developed intense flu symptoms, so I mixed some beautiful red hibiscus leaves with slippery elm, ginger, and mint, and made a strong herbal infusion by letting it steep for thirty minutes. I warned her that it was strong and may taste bitter, even with honey, and I suggested that she drink it slowly over the next two hours. Later in the class, she was excited to share that she felt better. This turned into a live demonstration on what herbs to use and how to process them for medicinal usage, and it reiterated why the Granny Midwives kept an herb garden, as do I.

Here are some herbs that Granny Midwives used for overall postpartum wellness:

- **Dandelion** (*Taraxacum officinale*) is a preventive, restorative adaptogen that aids the body in restoring its energy reserves. Grannies often instructed new mamas to drink a cup to get their body and energy back after birth. I mix one teaspoon dandelion leaf with one teaspoon peppermint and add honey. Dandelion is a common weed that grows in most yards. Along with making tea from the leaves, you can eat them by cooking them with your collards or turnip greens for a great source of iron.

- **Nettle** (*Urtica dioica*) is a great postpartum drink because of its high source of digestible iron and good quantity of calcium and vitamin A. These are essential vitamins and minerals for postpartum recuperation.

- **Lavender** (*Lavandula*) is suitable for aiding relaxation and helping with sleep. Mix a little lavender and coconut oils for a good postpartum foot massage.

- **Catnip** (*Nepeta cataria*) is good for easing postpartum cramping, nonspecific headaches, and infant colic. You can drink it warm with honey and a little lemon. When a postpartum mama feels restless, I like to give her a warm cup of mint mixed with catnip to help her relax and sleep.

- **Sassafras Bark** (*Sassafras albidum*) helps ease postpartum cramps. Use a small amount for a short period of time to avoid adverse effects.

- **Citrus fruits**, particularly lemons, oranges, and limes, became common as well. Midwives boiled them with honey and made a postpartum drink to build the new mom's immune system and prevent colds. It was common to enter a postpartum home and smell warm, tart citrus.

Note: Before you take any herbs, be sure to check with your healthcare provider to make sure you have no contraindications.

The Granny Midwife also knew that food was medicine, and nutritious meals would help new mothers heal well after birth. In the postpartum period, a new mother's family was provided certain meals that often included what is referred to today as "bone broth," made by slowly cooking greens with meat and its bones. Gumbo made with seafood and wild rice was a nourishing option, and watermelon juice, chicken liver, and beet leaves were also given after birth to build strength. On the other hand, there were certain foods that were taboo during the postpartum period. For example, many postpartum mothers were not allowed to eat pork or cabbage after birth, believing these foods inhibited proper digestion.[11]

Nutritious meals were so important to the health of postpartum families that every visitor was expected to bring enough food for the entire family when they visited the postpartum home. Beyond postpartum care, food was collectively understood to be a tasty method for healing, and Granny Midwives often invited folks to come by her home and get chicken eggs and greens from her garden to stay nourished.

As Michael Twitty writes in *The Cooking Gene*, "Black folks just knew that greens upheld life." Tender greens cooked down into a rich soup with some type of bone and meat added was a typical dish that recalls an ancestral African diet. Plenty of green, leafy vegetables and meat made for a hearty soup of protein and vitamins. Root vegetables, like turnips, beets, carrots, sweet potatoes, and sometimes a bowl of rice, would be added to provide extra sustenance and make sure mama felt full and content. Chicken soup was another popular meal. Chickens were easy to keep, so most people in the South kept them for their eggs and meat. A postpartum pot of chicken soup with a lot of yard vegetables, like onions, celery, tomatoes, and black-eyed peas, was both delicious and nutritious. Soft scrambled eggs in butter and gently seasoned with salt and pepper was an easy meal to provide that was good for mama.

The foods the new mama ate was offered to all in the household to eat, as postpartum food was family food, and most family members of age knew how to prepare the food for the new mother to keep her well fed after birth.

Return to Traditional African American Diet

It's important to return to the traditional African American diet because it will help you heal. I have witnessed plenty of mothers return to wellness by eating in this way. Know that food is medicine. You are what you eat. Eat the foods in their natural state the way the Creator intended. Make whole organic foods your first choice.

Herbal medicine is a universal healing method. It's simply wellness through plant life. Three-fourths of the world's population rely on herbal medicine, aka folk medicine, and prefer it over conventional medicine. Respect plant life as beautiful and healing because every plant has a different purpose. It is easier than you realize to incorporate these healing plants into your diet, as you likely already consume herbs regularly, whether you sprinkle dried parsley and chives on a meal, boil bay and basil leaves with your black-eyed-pea soup, or drink lavender tea to keep calm.

Spices are also a key part of our healing tool kit. The Granny Midwives believed that the internal system should never be sluggish because a sluggish inside creates health problems. They believed in generating heat by consuming hot foods with peppers, spicing with nutmeg, and drinking ginger tea, and using cinnamon and plenty of other spices in their recipes. These foods have a deep tradition in African American healing.

Some communities did not add heat and spice to their postpartum meals, but my family was notorious for adding small hot peppers to most of our dishes. Most of my grandmother's soups included hot peppers, white vinegar, and salt. My grandmother kept a bottle of white vinegar on the dining table with five hot peppers soaking inside, and after a few days, the vinegar would be so spicy, and we would pass it around to pour over our greens and to add flavor. Vinegar also aids in the body's ability to absorb calcium, which positively contributes to the healing of the uterus and pelvis.[12]

THE ERASURE OF THE GRANNY MIDWIFE

The practice of African American Granny Midwifery was eventually annihilated by laws and practices that discounted her contributions to her community and public health. As early as the 1910s, American public health professionals began to stigmatize Black midwives in a high-level campaign that the medical system labeled the "Midwife Problem."

The Granny Midwives often complained about how the white doctors would not come to help them when a Black mother had a problem with her birth, so to create discord and save their reputation, the public health system told pregnant families who had been using midwives since their arrival in America to no longer trust them. This woman, who had been a pillar of the community and respected by all, including the pastor, was now part of a smear campaign. The medical system told the community not to trust the Granny Midwife because she was old, dirty, ignorant, and dangerous. They did everything they could to discredit the Granny Midwife and pressure Black families into distancing themselves from her by saying things like, "She is uneducated. You are modern, and she is old-fashioned, and our way, the white way, is better."

This campaign was later legalized when the US Congress passed the National Maternity and Infancy Protection Act in November 1921, also called the Sheppard-Towner Act. This further reduced the practice of Granny Midwives by severely restricting their work and their ability to receive permits, allowing the public health department to force them into retirement. There are so many sad stories of dedicated and seasoned midwives arriving at their mandatory annual public health meeting to receive a cake and words of thanks for their work from outsiders. The community did not retire these midwives; outsiders did, and when a midwife went into retirement or a Granny Midwife was denied a new permit to continue practicing, they replaced her with white nurse midwives, thus ending the knowledge of African American postpartum care, beliefs, traditions, and rituals. All the while, influential physicians kept the assault going with claims that maternal and infant deaths persisted due to the lack of midwifery regulation and unskilled midwives. However, this was later proven untrue.[13] Most doctors were not interested in working with Black midwives or assisting Black birthing and postpartum mothers. Sadly, studies as recent as 2022 show the same attitude.

By the 1930s, most Southern states had ended the right for Granny Midwives to renew their permits, which were required for them to legally practice as midwives. Without a permit, the midwives would be arrested if they continued to serve their pregnant families with home birth and postpartum care.

Black physicians also had to buy into the white medical model and distance themselves from Granny Midwives, who may have been their church members. But because Black doctors were educated and licensed by the dominant culture, they had no options. They needed to be in good standing with the white medical establishment to be successful as physicians. In 1941, the Historically Black College and University (HBCU) Tuskegee School of Nurse-Midwifery was founded. Its purpose was to train younger African American women who were literate and had assimilated into Western medicine.[14] At Tuskegee, students learned to rebuff the ways of the Granny Midwives and their traditional practices.[15] The Tuskegee School of Nurse-Midwifery only lasted for five years, from 1941–1946.

The systemic distancing and attack of the Granny Midwife and the discounting of her years of service gradually pushed Black pregnant women to white male medical care, which knew nothing of Black birthing traditions, postpartum care rituals, or African-centered newborn care. It took fifty years of brutal propaganda to dissolve our traditions in a community that was cohesive, tight-knit, and knew what was expected to achieve wellness for a new mother, baby, and the community after birth.[16] The African American community experienced emotional and social trauma in the eradication of the Granny Midwife.

This was a dark time in US history, increasing the legacy of injustices that continue today for Black women.[17] Today, African American women have disproportionately higher rates of postpartum morbidity and mortality, even as the Centers for Disease Control and Prevention (CDC) states that 60 percent of these deaths are preventable. Acknowledging and returning to the Granny

Midwife's postpartum traditions and rituals is one way to reclaim our culture, safeguard our postpartum health, master our recuperation, and uplift ourselves as beautiful Black mothers. When we lost our Granny Midwife, we lost her healing, warmth, familiarity, love, and holistic nourishment in our postpartum period.

We Will Remember

As a new mother, remember the love of our Granny Midwives and honor their legacy by practicing the African American postpartum tradition of deeply resting after birth for forty-two days, eating soups, staying warm, and not fearing motherhood because we know that motherhood and babies are sacred gifts from the Creator.

AN UNBROKEN LINK TO CULTURAL KNOWLEDGE

Like James Brown once said, "Say it loud: I am Black, and I am proud." I am a proud Black woman, and I am the proud bearer of our traditions. As a descendant of African-born midwives, the Granny Midwife was the link in maintaining the remnants of African cultural knowledge of postpartum care, newborn care, and motherhood. She upheld the Black family's links to their ancestral birth traditions and postpartum rituals, the divinity of motherhood, the honor and love of fatherhood, and the spirituality that taught communal support. She was respected for her knowledge and healing skills, her ability to bring peace to any situation, and her wisdom in solving problems. She was a protector of the postpartum mother, ensuring that the mother could rest, nurse her baby, and fully recover from her birth;

and she helped women who wanted to practice the African midwifery ways as their mothers and grandmothers did. She kept the postpartum traditions alive and was an avid defender and keeper of the culture that had been brought from Africa to America.[18]

The Granny Midwife acted with love, guidance, skill, spirituality, and family-strengthening techniques. She honored the beauty of the Black woman, reminding us that Black skin, in its various shades, is normal and beautiful and teaching us how to care for it as new mothers with African beautification ceremonies. She also celebrated and supported healthy male/female relationships.[19]

I have always had a longing in my heart to know the truth about Black culture. Once I became a midwife, my postpartum education allowed me to feel pride in knowing that my culture cared deeply and completely for the new mother and her newborn, using ancient ways with a proven track record of honoring new mothers and bringing their bodies, minds, and spirits back to equilibrium. I say equilibrium because I learned that the Granny Midwives taught that, after birth, women's bodies are open and susceptible to illness. The lying-in period allows the mother's body to return to balance through various ancestral traditions, like those I've touched on in this chapter.

For years, I served families after birth and taught budding midwives and doulas what I learned. They were grateful to have access to the ways of the Granny Midwives and learn their words of encouragement, herbal formulas, soups, teas, and taboos that would protect the mother from getting ill. Mainly, I retrieved the loving way of our ancestors, who holistically cared for the new mother and honored her with prayer and positive affirmations. Their template was one of multidimensional care, which helped women heal and transform into motherhood by way of nurturance, nourishment, intimacy, and warmth.

What I found in the Granny Midwives was a needed philosophy, the foundation of Black postpartum care, and the knowledge that the Black community needs to know for empowerment, pride, connection, confidence, and health. This was the way of the Granny Midwife, whose Motherwit, community care, and natural healing knowledge celebrated and honored Black motherhood and Black babies. These ways are no longer hidden; they are here, waiting for us to reclaim them.

We reclaim our rights to health with gratitude to the Granny Midwives, who understood that motherhood is a positive physical and spiritual experience. We reclaim our African American roots, which tell us that motherhood is a blessing. And though motherhood comes with many challenges, we know how to resolve them and find relief. We reclaim our joy in being mothers! Believe in your cultural ways and learn how to practice the traditions and rituals in this book for full postpartum recuperation and a peaceful mind. The African American postpartum culture has been retrieved as our birthright. Claim your postpartum traditions and regain your strength in all areas, including your faith and confidence in yourself to be a good mother.

CHAPTER 2

Sankofa: Stirring Up Healing Traditions

Bless the ones who went back to reclaim our postpartum traditions for healing the new mother and protecting the newborn. Bless those who now maintain these traditions and pass them on to future generations. Sankofa is our birthright to go back and fetch from the past. Knowing our past and learning from it helps us heal and honor our ancestors and the generations to come. It brightens our future with relevant knowledge for all things, particularly African American postpartum traditions.

ON AUGUST 23, 1976, I WOKE UP TO THE CRIES OF MY NEWBORN SON. Instinctively, I picked him up and nursed him. He eventually fell back to sleep, so I laid him down and took a warm shower. After my shower, I realized I was hungry and had not eaten anything during my eighteen hours of labor at home. The doctor and my support person left a couple of hours after my homebirth, and neither advised me of when or what to eat. I remember pouring cereal and milk into a bowl and eating it in front of the television. After eating my bowl of cereal, I called to let my family and friends know that I had given birth to a baby boy.

Though everyone congratulated me over the phone, I knew something was missing. I was happy to have my baby, but looking back, I can see that there was no joy or celebration in my postpartum period. No one came to check on me or bring me food, and no one came to beautify me. My friends were my age, eighteen to twenty-one years old, and we did not know what we were supposed to do for one another after the birth of a baby. When my husband and I decided to have our first child at home, there was nothing for me to read about Black postpartum traditions.

When my niece was born, I remember my mother mentioning things like not bringing the baby out of the house until after the cord fell off, not going out with the baby on cold days, and keeping socks and hats on a newborn when leaving the house, no matter the weather. But she passed away when I was fifteen. If she had been alive, I know she would have celebrated me as a new mother and loved on her new grandbaby. She would have cared for me using our ancestral healing traditions. She would have gathered family and friends and announced that her grandbaby had arrived and that her daughter had safely given birth. She would have said, "Now, come over and help care for her," because caring for the new mama is part of the celebration.

To ensure that future generations understand the ancestral ways of caring for themselves and others, as well as being cared for by others, we need an instructional blueprint on how and why certain things are done during the postpartum period. That blueprint exists in the African American postpartum culture that prioritizes the well-being of both mother and baby. These traditions activate and elevate our culture and help make full postpartum recuperation accessible to all. Now, we need to reclaim them.

Going back to reclaim our traditions is a form of Sankofa. An Adinkra symbol of the Akan people of the region now known as Ghana, Sankofa is represented by a large bird with its head facing backward and an egg held in its beak. Sankofa means to go back and reclaim lost knowledge, to recover and fetch the truth from the past. A deeper meaning is that it is not taboo to go back and get what was forgotten; in fact, it is expected that we do.

To me, it means we are unapologetic in reclaiming our African American postpartum ways, regardless of the time and place in history. The door of the past remains open to retrieve forgotten or stolen information. Sankofa allows us to return to our way of caring for postpartum women and newborns—a way that builds up our humanity so we can nurture ourselves and our babies. This book is, itself, a practice of Sankofa, holding the traditions we have retrieved.

Our past traditions are nothing short of a miracle; they are the healing for today and the future. Our ancient medicine quiets the mind after a long birth, allows the body to be still so the organs can return to their prepregnant state, and helps the spirit reflect gratitude. The ancestors say you can't move forward if you don't know your past. By keeping an eye on our history, we become confident, prideful, and powerful as we grow into the beautiful role of a mother: to nurture and receive. Our history reminds us how to sustain ourselves by valuing family and community, an integral part of healing. Reclaiming our past is our responsibility and right to know ourselves and all the great things we have done to honor mothers and cherish our babies. With Sankofa, you go back and get what you need to be whole, which is the beginning of a full postpartum recovery.

Practicing Sankofa with Elders and Children
I went back to fetch our African American postpartum traditions to elevate the health of Black women after their birth. I

hope this book is part of your practice of Sankofa as well as a catalyst for you to fetch more and more of our traditions from history and your own life, families, and communities. With the Granny Midwives as our touchstone, we can keep looking—in written accounts, oral histories, and passed-down traditions and rituals. When we do this, we are learning from the past to make better decisions in the future.

When you are fetching past knowledge, consider asking everyone you know for stories of what they have seen, heard, or were told by their elders or knowledgeable peers. Talk with your elders, as they have gained much wisdom through their lived experiences, which gives them the ability to share outcomes from healthy traditions. They are also closer to the past to recall what postpartum care looked like in their time of history.

You can also practice Sankofa by teaching your children how to help a new mother. The African style of care has always been communal, so even young children knew their role. The youth jobs, from ages four to ten, included holding the baby, changing diapers, dressing the baby, bringing the new mama a plate of food or taking her soiled plates to the kitchen, bringing her a cup of water, getting things that she asked for, or bringing messages from grandma, such as "Granny asked if you wanted another blanket." These roles were taught by way of observation, expectation, and the cultural belief that helping those in need was service work for God. And it was expected that the older children would show the younger children how to help. We need to fetch this tradition of teaching children to understand and respect the postpartum time and their role in ensuring that the new mother and baby thrive.

Don't forget the men. I have gained so much wisdom speaking to men who took care of their mother, wife, or daughter during the postpartum period. Many women have told me that their dad was the healer of the family, and he took care of them after the birth of their babies. I love hearing those testimonials.

One of the core values of our traditions is that motherhood is sacred and honorable. It is okay to implement the foundation of our traditions in a way that works best for you and your family; no matter how you practice our traditions, it should reflect compassionate and empowering ways of honoring the mother.

HONORING THE RICHNESS OF OUR TRADITIONS

The exciting part for me is seeing all the variation in our traditions because, like all cultures that have subcultures, clans, faith house traditions, and families, beliefs within African American culture are not a monolith. African American postpartum traditions are influenced by geographic location; what foods, herbs, and other resources were most available in that region; people's religious beliefs; and what remnants of traditions were maintained and passed on from different parts of Africa. Even the Granny Midwife may not have known why the lying-in period was three months in her community, but two months for families who lived fifty miles away. It may have been influenced by another African culture, as a mix of ethnic groups were brought to America.

Over the years, I have documented oral histories from women all over the United States, from the seashore of the Gullah Islands to rural Alabama, the mountains of Tennessee, inner cities on the East Coast, arid deserts, and more. Women from the Gullah were told to refrain from eating cabbage and greens for the first few weeks after birth, but they were fed tons of seafood gumbo with beans and rice. Women from Alabama told me they couldn't go past the front gate for six weeks post-birth, they had to keep their head covered, and they could not bring the baby outside for weeks. A woman from Florida told me they weren't allowed to eat pork for the first month after the birth. Others explained that they couldn't sit on the side of the bed and swing their legs for fear of blood clots being let loose, while others said that the women of the house took turns sleeping with the baby to allow the mother to sleep at night.

Going back and fetching this information is emotional for me because I see our history replaying in my mind, and I can imagine what it was like to be in a home with family members and close neighbors who knew how to care for a new mother and her baby. They were available and willing to care for the mother, and the mother did not worry or stress because she knew she had an entire army of caretakers. In contrast, many of today's mothers are so worried about how they're going to care for themselves and their baby that they can't properly relax and they don't feel safe. This contributes to chronic stress, which can impact the immune system and increase the chances of maternal morbidity, exhaustion, and postpartum depression.

Reclaiming our postpartum traditions and rituals also involves learning about rural Black Southern traditions and their links to African culture. I focused much of my initial research on the rural South because, due to segregation, Black people had more time and space to practice their traditional African ways without outside influence. In fact, up until the late 1930s, Black people had maintained many African-based postpartum traditions, including belly binding, newborn waist beads, low lighting for rest, selective diets, protective prayers, and rituals to prevent postpartum problems.

We can trace the variations between the original traditions and the need to improvise through our different locales, each with their own seasonal patterns and native foods. Just as we see the connection between certain African American foods and our African origins, such as the New Orleans red beans and rice with the red-bean soup of Zanzibar, we can begin to see connections between our grandmothers' postpartum care and the way particular African cultures care for their newborns and mothers.

THE ANTIDOTE TO THE WESTERN MEDICAL MODEL

If you've picked up this book, you're probably well aware that today's medical model of birth and postpartum care has had a negative influence on how we practice our cultural postpartum traditions, both physically and psychologically, especially in how we embrace motherhood. The Western model depicts motherhood as a negative experience and even as a burden. This is the opposite of African American mothering philosophy, where motherhood is normal and viewed as a badge of honor and grandeur. For generations now, as Virginian midwife and author of *The Life and Time of a Virginia Midwife* Claudine Curry Smith put it, young people believed in what the doctors said and did not practice African American postpartum care.[1] This made it hard for them to participate in their own recuperation, mainly because they stopped listening to the elders and did not understand the dos and don'ts of their cultural postpartum care.

THE DEFINITION OF THE POSTPARTUM PERIOD

The Western medical definition of the postpartum period is the first six weeks after birth, during which pregnancy hormone levels return to their nonpregnant state and the reproductive organs return to their prepregnant size and location in the pelvis. During this time, doctors typically check new mothers' vital signs, such as blood pressure, temperature, weight, and pulse; observe the healing of their vaginal tissue after an episiotomy; check for a contracted uterus and excessive bleeding; and complete a mental health screening to detect postpartum depression.

Standard Western postpartum care has a scant schedule of visits, with just two recommended, at three and six weeks postpartum, unless there are medical problems, such as an infection from a cesarean section. At six weeks, women who had vaginal births are usually cleared to have sex and engage in normal daily activities, whereas in African American postpartum care, six weeks of abstinence and rest is the minimum. Basically, the Western medical message is *everything is done; now get back to your normal life.*

The Western postpartum model of care emphasizes physical and mental risks. It prescribes antidepressants for postpartum depression and strongly recommends birth control. It confirms that you can expect to feel exhausted and overwhelmed and suffer from a variety of maladies, such as painful sex, incontinence, body aches, and a colicky baby. At her postpartum clinic visits, rarely does a mother get a congratulations; she isn't reassured that everything is going to be fine, and that with each week, she will begin to feel stronger and more confident in her mothering and decision-making. Mamas aren't told, "You can have a full life as a mother; it is not one or the other."

On top of this, Black women also get the subtle and overt message that they don't deserve to be a mother. Instead of getting congratulations from the medical community during our prenatal visits or postpartum visits, new Black mothers are often asked what birth control they are using. In addition, the medical community suggests that Black women are generally unhealthy and should not be having babies, saying that by virtue of being Black, we are automatically high risk, linking this to the high Black maternal mortality, when these deaths are actually a result of systemic racism. There's even the government-waged propaganda that Black women only have babies to get welfare checks, when in reality most Black women return to work within two weeks postpartum to avoid needing welfare. Because of this propaganda, some women feel like failures being home all day with their baby because society does not view motherhood as a valid job, even though we know it is. In fact, in recent years, a new term has emerged to support stay-at-home mothers and validate the hard work it takes to care for herself, her children, and her household: "domestic engineers."

As a mother of seven children, I remember the negative responses I received from the medical community and, unfortunately, my own community, even though I was doing it "right," according to societal standards. I was over the age of eighteen, college-educated, married, and employed, and I was still treated like I was doing something wrong. People would try to shame me by saying things like, "Don't you know about birth control?" "How many more are you going to have?" or "Don't ask me to babysit." Fortunately, I knew their responses were the result of years of harmful stereotypes against Black women, but it didn't help it sting any less. Black fathers also bear the brunt of this, being told that it is irresponsible to bring another child into the world, being reminded that kids are expensive, or being asked how they will manage the added responsibility or assumed lack of a sex life.

There is an ongoing attack on the Black family, including the forced sterilization of Black women in the United States and around the globe, poor pregnancy support from medical institutions and society at large, and the myth of overpopulated Black communities ruining the environment.

All this negativity during pregnancy can weigh poorly on the postpartum experience. If you have been stressed by implicit bias for your entire pregnancy, then expect that you may need to do a lot of unpacking after birth. Many women have told me how much the medical system stressed them out during their prenatal care by telling them that their baby was not healthy and continuously recommending them to terminate their pregnancy, even after they declined. They would tell me that by the time the baby was born, they were a nervous wreck and could barely relax. They had become hypervigilant in their postpartum period, overly worrying about every little thing.

These are just some of the reasons Sankofa is so important and powerful for Black families during the prenatal and postpartum periods. Black families are powerful, strong, and beautiful. Supporting Black mothers and fathers is not only a way to ensure the health of the individual family, but to overturn the Western messages that have maligned us. I love to see the smiles on parents' faces when they meet their new baby, and I always make it a point to congratulate them. They always light up at this simple gesture. Imagine if new parents were congratulated all day from strangers who walked by. What would that do for their mental health? Perhaps postpartum depression wouldn't be as severe or last as long.

Our traditions insist on valuing the mother. Instituting this would reduce the number of women who feel the need to rush back into the workforce, not for money, but to assert that they are a productive member of society. We can help diminish the ambivalence in becoming or being a mother by lovingly mothering the mother through our traditions. Motherhood should be validated and viewed as one of the ultimate professions because mothers employ many skills and techniques to support the growth and health of their children and, in turn, the future of society.

The Heavy Weight

I have noticed that in the Western postpartum care model, mamas are expected to take their newborn to numerous pediatric appointments to discuss things like colic, sleep, feeding schedules, weight gain, and immunizations, all while carrying a fifty-pound car seat, with baby, her purse, and a baby bag. And no one helps her! She is on her own! I frequently point out this abnormality in my doula training and when speaking to families and the public. On one hand, medical professionals advise new mothers to not lift anything heavier than the baby for the first month, yet the mother is often forced to carry everything to a doctor's appointment and when shopping. This excess weight can cause long-term damage to the mother's skeleton, which has not yet stabilized from relaxin, the hormone that makes the pelvis mobile enough for the baby to pass through during birth.

In my presentations and consultations, I remind family and friends to be there for the new mother and carry the car seat and extra bags for her. I also recommend new mamas to carry just the baby and not the car seat. It is better for her body and the baby's emotional and physical health because the more the baby is in physical contact with their mother, the warmer they'll stay, the better they'll bond, and the more opportunities there will be for organic feeding, which ensures healthy weight gain. Please leave the car seat in the car, and just carry the baby for the first six months.

WE MOTHER THE MOTHER

The African American postpartum tradition offers a holistic approach because so much is happening simultaneously, both physically and emotionally, during the postpartum period. It's more than reproductive organs settling after pregnancy; it's also digestion and skin changes, breast engorgement, bleeding, hormonal fluctuations, pelvic floor changes, and so much more—not to mention the new intense emotions you'll feel for your new baby! Many mothers are surprised by the intensity of love they feel.

For this reason, the African American postpartum period includes physical, emotional, and spiritual healing as well as medical support as needed. It prioritizes social support from family, friends, midwives, and doulas who come to help and celebrate the new family unit. I often share a variety of important reminders with new mamas: "Get back in bed," "It is expected to feel tired; you had a baby two weeks ago," and "Vaginal discomfort can last up to eight weeks and longer sometimes; keep taking your postpartum baths." It is a time of transformation and learning, of bonding and healing.

Our traditions emphasize warm, nourishing foods, mainly soups, stews, and tonics, as well as prayers and herbs to help restore the mother from the inside out. We emphasize loving and nurturing the mother, supporting her body and emotions with natural remedies, and employing community care to prevent or quickly remedy common postpartum concerns. We honor the postpartum period with the patience needed to allow new mothers to feel supported.

You Are Worthy of Care
The concept of mothering the mother is the heart of this care. This means, in part, that you must believe you are cared for by

someone who will be there for you, whether it's your mother or a mother figure.[2] When a Granny Midwife said, "Go lay or sit down," most new mothers would respect that and abide. It's important for you to know that you are worthy of this kind of mothering and mother care. You will likely need help practicing rest, embracing the concept of self-love, and accepting care, service, and celebration from your caretakers. You will need to get comfortable with human touch to receive massages with warm healing oils, like sesame, coconut oil, and shea butter, and postpartum herbal baths. You will need help embracing the ancient spiritual practices of postpartum care, such as prayer, affirmation, meditation, and song, and allow loved ones to lay hands on you. These healing practices are critical to counteract the victimization of Black motherhood by the media, which tends to end with sad news of death and illness. Not true. African American postpartum care speaks to the resilience and wholeness of healing and our legacy of living, thriving, and reproducing ourselves for a better tomorrow.

We must be authentic in our culture of mothering the mother and learn how to heal during postpartum to emerge from the transformation of birth as healthy, vibrant, and empowered mothers. The postpartum period is a rite of passage in the African American tradition, one that is necessary to restore your strength and protect your newborn against illness. There is always discomfort during rites of passage, but when you are fully supported in it, you will experience emotional and intellectual growth. This is why mothers are so respected in African and African American culture because they have become confident within themselves. It is a beautiful thing! We acknowledge and honor that this sacred passage is made of caring rituals for the mother and the newborn that include the extended family and the community, whose purpose is to surround the new family with help, love, healing herbs, wisdom, and nutritious foods. The goal is to always prioritize the mother and infant's wellness and happiness.

Our postpartum traditions show us that motherhood is not a burden, but a beautiful and sacred act, a blessing. African Americans' belief in the divinity of motherhood is built into African American spirituality and the high values we have always placed on family and children.[3] The Granny Midwives said time and again that the work of serving birthing mothers was God's work, and you had to have patience, kindness, and humor to help them regain their physical strength and be confident in motherhood. These same attributes carry over into providing postpartum nurturing.

After birth, mothers can feel weak and cold inside. This is why a big part of our postpartum traditions is focused on helping the new mother become strong and maintain her warmth. This not only helps her body heal, but it restores the warmth of her spirit and helps reintegrate it back into the physical realm. Our culture recognizes that birth is both normal and a profound spiritual experience, in which the mother's soul leaves her body to bring forth life from the spirit realm. The postpartum period is when the work is done to stabilize her spirit in her body with intentional rituals and regimens. If the new mother is not nourished immediately and consistently, she will feel depleted and disconnected from her baby and body. This is why our traditions focus so much on preventing these postpartum morbidities by honoring and celebrating motherhood with our traditions of prayer, warmth, cleansing, nutrition, hydration, herbs, rest, family support, commune, and love. You are worthy of this care, and you are doing our ancestors a great service by reclaiming these traditions.

FATHERING THE FATHER

In twentieth-century African American culture, it was the women, the matriarchs of the family, who primarily provided postpartum care, but over the last twenty years or so, Western cultures and the prevalence of the nuclear family has shifted the responsibility of postpartum care from grandmothers and female family and community members to the spouse or baby's father. Dads are now expected to have increased involvement in the birth of their babies and offer more hands-on help to support the health of both mother and baby. To this end, more and more states have begun offering paid paternal leave so fathers can be involved in the birth and help during those early postpartum weeks.

Although we can point to changes in societal norms and roles for this shift in postpartum caretakers, this is also partly the result of female members not being available to help, the growing family living far from their extended family system, or a lack of family friends. In addition, Black men today have a better understanding of just how much rest a new mother needs to heal, and unfortunately the Black maternal mortality rate has put more Black men on alert to provide postpartum care as a way to protect the new mother from maternal morbidity and mortality. Over the years, many more fathers have asked me what they can do to help, and they are often eager to attend childbirth classes to be knowledgeable on birth and the postpartum experience.

While it's necessary for us to talk at length about caring for mother and baby, it's important to also include fathers in conversations about postpartum care. When my son's partner went into labor, I was blessed to be at the birth of my grandchild and watch my son catch his daughter. A few hours after the birth, the maternal grandmother arrived. It was our first time meeting, and we hit it off. Being pretty much of the same generation and Southern culture, we both knew why we were there: to mother the mother, honor the father, and help care for the new grandbaby. There were three of us there to help the mother, and us two grandmothers frequently relieved Dad so he could rest, enjoy his new baby, and love on his woman.

I would prepare the postpartum bathwater, the maternal grandmother would prepare meals, and the dad would hold his baby so mama could rest, occasionally running errands for the house. On the third day postpartum, the maternal grandma and I cooked an elaborate breakfast: grits, chicken and gravy, finely chopped turnip greens, and soft scrambled eggs with sautéed onions, cream cheese, and a hot chili sauce. We also made sweet red raspberry, ginger, nettle, and mint herbal drinks to benefit the new mother, although the father had a cup to drink as well. I made two breakfast plates and presented the food on a beautiful tray to the mother and father, who both were in bed with their baby in the middle. When I served them their food, I remember my son saying, "If I am going to be treated like a king, then let's keep having babies."

I love sharing this story because it demonstrates how we can practice African American postpartum care and celebrate both the mother and father in the process. The father should feel included, acknowledged, fed, and supported as well.

At the same time, there are spouses or partners who don't provide help after birth for a variety of reasons: They don't believe it is their job, they don't know how to help, or work takes them away from the house for long periods of time, which is often the case for truck drivers, firefighters, the military, and other professions. I have also helped many postpartum mothers who broke up with the father of their baby early in their pregnancy. Circumstances may vary, but one thing I want to see is fathers learning and embracing African American postpartum traditions. They should know what the postpartum period is, why their support is essential, and that they deserve relief breaks, when possible. This will help new fathers feel supported so they can find their place in their fatherhood.

A Prayer for Fathers

Dear God,

Bless this new father (baba). May he have a loving relationship with his new baby, may he have intuition to support the new mother, may he have gratitude for the blessing of family, may he be prosperous in caring for and protecting his family, and may he be blessed with good health and a long life. Send him help in the sacred postpartum period so he may experience the blessings of African American postpartum traditions and rituals.

Fathers, if you feel overwhelmed, please ask for help. It is not a sign of weakness but rather a sign of strength. Remember the African proverb, "It takes a village." Congratulations on being a father!

LYING-IN

Though birth is beautiful, it is a physical and emotional experience that takes an enormous amount of energy. The goal is to use the lying-in period to bring new mothers back to wellness while supporting them in bonding with their newborn. Traditionally, the lying-in period is the first and most intensive postpartum phase, about forty-two days long. Since it takes six weeks for the uterus to shrink and find its correct place within the pelvis, I consider this a critical time. The ritual of lying-in is the protective factor for a continuously positive postpartum experience beyond the first six weeks. The entire African American postpartum period takes longer, usually from six months to a year or more, and can include everything from parenting advice to potty training help to relationship support. But that initial lying-in period encompasses those crucial first six weeks after the birth of a baby. As we've discussed, this is when the new mother needs consistent mothering, with restorative postpartum meals, consideration, advice, and love. This period supports her in developing her sense of accomplishment, confidence, and gratitude so she can learn and accept what she needs to in this new phase of life and graciously grow into her motherhood.

Listen to Black Mothers

SisterSong Women of Color Reproductive Justice Collective, an activist organization in Atlanta, Georgia, that works to reduce poor maternal outcomes, argues that Black women are often not taken seriously or heard when they say something is wrong. We must practice Sankofa and go back and fetch the tradition of listening to Black mamas. The Granny Midwife was wise. She listened to the new mother with empathy and no judgment. When a new mother said, "I am not connecting to my baby. I didn't want this baby, and I feel so alone," she would listen and ask what she needed. She'd then offer the traditions and rituals she knew could help the new mama manage her postpartum challenges. We all need to listen to Black mothers, as they are the experts of their situation. You are the expert.

As a midwife, I often made postpartum visits, only to find that most moms were alone because their spouse was at work, their own mother was coming to help in a few weeks, or they simply didn't have a supportive community. I remember the most enjoyable part of the postpartum visit for new moms was after I had checked their vital signs and saw that everything was progressing normally. I would sit, have a cup of tea with them, and socialize with them for ten to fifteen minutes. When it was time for me to leave, many of them would say, "I feel so much better," or they'd ask, "When is our next visit?" New mothers need visitors who know how to sit, listen, help, and not overstay their welcome so they can get back to resting.

FUSSING

"Fussing" is also central to the lying-in period. Fussing means "to give attention, shower with attention, or hover over with concern." As a midwife, my focus is always on the mother, as she is the most important person in the room. Many of the rituals you'll see in the following pages are ways to fuss over you as a new mother. The goal is to help you feel beautiful, special, cared about, and loved. We fuss during the lying-in with rituals of beauty, health, and prosperity to bring you joy and hope, help you heal from birth, and strengthen you from the inside out.

> ### *Healing at Any Time*
> *The Creator made the female a goddess who can birth life and heal herself at any time with the right tools. While the first forty-two days of postpartum is the foundation of long-term recuperation, everything in this book can be used for healing and uplifting, no matter how long you've been postpartum. I once worked with the mother of a two-year-old who was not given the traditional lying-in period when her baby was born, and as a result, she had a very traumatic early postpartum period. I encouraged her to practice the rituals, baths, and dietary advice, even though it had been years since her birth. She was amazed by how much her emotional state improved and how much more confident she felt as a mother. It's never too late! You can practice these rituals at any time, and I especially recommend doing so if you were never given this kind of care when your baby was a newborn.*

COMMUNAL CARE

Don't let challenges prevent you from caring for yourself. Although times have changed and many of us have smaller extended families, live farther away from family members, lack postpartum traditional knowledge, have to return to work soon after birth, do not have consistent access to maternity and paternity leave, and are generally overstimulated by the society we live in, we still must find ways to practice African American postpartum care on our terms because we deserve it.

The African concept of "we," and not the Western concept of "I," is the heart and soul of African American postpartum traditions.

The focus is on the mother and baby together and the family and community at large because we think collectively and believe that healing is a communal act. African American postpartum care, though woman-centered, is also inclusive of male/female experiences, as what affects the mother could affect the new father, and vice versa. Granny Midwives honored and helped the father too, giving him a listening ear, empathy, and suggestions to address the challenges he may be experiencing as a new father and protector of the mother.

Everyone is responsible for caring for the mother, baby, and family unit. In our tradition, postpartum care is a continuum of support, though it will look different over the months and years to come. I always suggest that moms and families organize their support early so mama can fully inhabit the lying-in period and take it slow. In the second and third postpartum months, moms need help with taking naps, getting massages, taking care of the baby, and breastfeeding. Familial titles like Grandma, Nana, Auntie, Grandpa, Uncle, Sister, and Brother highlight the notion that everyone has a responsibility to act in motherly and fatherly ways to support the family and offer relief to the mother.

This emphasis on community also requires you, as a new mother, to ask for help when you need it and accept it when it's offered. This is in direct contrast to our current era, where being independent is considered strong and asking for help is considered weak. This can be the breaking point for your positive postpartum recuperation. If you feel like you need to figure it out alone or isolate after birth, you are not indulging in our ancestral postpartum care structure, which is inherently communal. Instead, plan for lots of community support, and remember that it is okay to ask for help. You deserve it.

BUILDING COMMUNITY SUPPORT

Every new mother deserves and needs postpartum support. Research shows that immediate support after birth reduces postpartum illnesses, such as heavy bleeding, headaches, and postpartum depression.[4] We are high-level mammals that were created for interpersonal interaction. This is why the African American postpartum tradition encourages family and community participation. The new mom should have at least one woman in the house with her at all times, even if the baby's father is present. Even better if there are a multitude of responsible people around to prevent her from feeling lonely or unsupported during this critical time. Consistent care over an extended period is needed for new mothers to regain their strength of mind, body, and spirit, and this is a community effort. But what do you do when there is no spousal or immediate family support?

I challenge you to pick up the African American postpartum tradition of asking neighbors and friends for help. If there are no partners, family, or friends, then you need to navigate how to get the help you deserve. You need to know that you deserve to be cared for after you have a baby. Regardless of the story behind your pregnancy, you are a queen. It is your birthright. As a Black woman, you must reclaim your postpartum culture. Remember, the Granny Midwives and community eagerly waited on us hand and foot after we had our babies. They mothered and cared for us so we would be healthy and happy. You need this now.[5]

Please don't think you must be independent and go it alone. That is not our culture. Reach out to your cousins and friends whom you might not have spoken to for years and ask for their help during your postpartum period. Contact your in-laws and ask if they can come over at least once a day or whenever they can. Make a schedule in advance so you know what support is available to you.

If you still have no help, reach out to social programs like Healthy Start. Let the patient advocate at your hospital know that you are looking for physical help during your postpartum period, hire a postpartum doula, sign up for a postpartum meal train service, or look into hiring a student midwife or doula who needs postpartum hours for their graduation. Look into online communities and support groups at hospitals, faith houses, and community organizations. Try to have your schedule prepared by the time you're five to eight months pregnant.

Lastly, cook up three to five meals from the recipe section of this book and freeze them so they are ready for your postpartum journey. If you're in a pinch and need an easy, nutritious meal after birth, you can throw onions, celery, carrots, a bag of precut collards, and a whole chicken in a crockpot; cover the chicken with water; add a half teaspoon of salt, a broken bay leaf, two teaspoons of garlic powder, one teaspoon of cayenne pepper; cover and go lay back down until it is cooked. Once it's ready after an hour or two, take what you want to eat from the pot, then put the rest in the fridge. You can always warm up some more the next day.

Tips for Creating Ease

While nothing substitutes community care, there are things you can do to prepare and create more ease for yourself:

Meals: Use disposable dishes or one dedicated ceramic bowl that you wash after each use. Ensure that everyone in the family eats the same food—yes, even children. No cooking a bunch of separate meals.

Rest: *Small toddlers sleep in your room on blankets on the floor or in a sleeping bag. If needed, everyone can camp out together in the front room to better serve your needs.*

Let your children help: *If you have children, teach them to help before the baby is born. The Granny Midwife was known for teaching children how to help and what to do. Again, it is an honor and a privilege for everyone in the family to wait on the postpartum mother, so teach your children that this is their culture, and they are blessed to help their mother and new sibling be healthy. Please don't feel guilty about this. I had all my children help with each of their new siblings, regardless of their age. They changed diapers, washed dishes, made me tea, and some even cooked and held the baby while I did something I wanted to do. I made sure that each of them is qualified to walk into any postpartum home and help, and I instilled in them that they are blessed to serve postpartum mothers.*

Schedule assistance: *At the end of the book, you will find a calendar you can use to help your support system sign up for the days they will visit and the activities they'll do to help. This way, if your family knows nothing about what postpartum care entails yet they still want to help, the tasks are listed for you. Try not to worry about how your house looks. I'd advise taking the garbage out right before you give birth; otherwise everything else can wait until your forty-two-day lying-in period is over.*

In African spirituality, babies are our gift from God, and to show gratitude for that gift, everyone is responsible for taking care of the mother and the newborn.

RETURNING TO WHOLENESS

Our culture knows it is a blessing to bring forth new life, and it is the community's job to protect the new mother from hostile outside forces, such as sad and shocking news and physically demanding household chores. As we reclaim our postpartum traditions, we must embrace the core goal of protecting the new mother and her baby so they can heal and bond with each other and the father. Remember, healing takes time. It is a slow process for a good reason. Just go with.

Our traditions show that a well-cared-for mother has the best chance of a full postpartum recovery and a thriving infant. When we ensure that new mothers regain their strength and stamina, we center the whole person. Mothering the mother has seven key principles that should be practiced daily during the lying-in period and continued regularly throughout the entire postpartum time:

1. Honor and Prayer
Prayer and respect for the living is our foundation of healing.

We believe in our connection to, and faith in, the universal life force, which creates the whole and manifests with prayer as the new mother's complete postpartum recuperation and the newborn's health. We say the prayer of the Granny Midwives of Mississippi: "Our heavenly father, the author and finishers of our life, we give thanks for health and strength and all the joys of life. We ask that you bless the mothers and fathers everywhere and make them more loving in what they say and do."

2. Warmth
Warming yourself both inside and out heals the body, the emotions, and the spirit.

Heat is essential for postpartum healing. Warmth helps postpartum mothers feel embraced, relaxed, and rejuvenated, as heat increases oxygen to the needed areas of the body.

3. Cleanliness
We cleanse for hygiene, healing, and energetic clarity.

The mantra "Cleanliness is next to Godliness" is a public health imperative to prevent postpartum infection. Being and feeling clean enhances the mood, promotes healing, and allows new mothers to engage with the element of water, which is a powerful energetic source.

4. Nourishment
A nourished mother is a healthy mother.

During the postpartum period, we focus on replenishing the nutrients used during pregnancy, labor, and birth to prevent postpartum depletion and build strength.

5. Herbal Healing and Hydration
Medicinal herbs and plenty of water will replenish and sustain you.

Herbs are gentle yet powerful ways to heal, nourish, and beautify the body. One excellent way to use herbs is to drink them through infusions because it helps new mothers stay hydrated while their body heals from the herbs' medicinal benefits.

6. Rest
You deserve to rest.

Rest is the foundation of African American postpartum care. This is why the lying-in period focuses so heavily on sleeping, relaxing, and rejuvenating.

7. Love

We encircle the mother and her baby with positive vibrations.

The basis of postpartum care is love, no matter the number of pregnancies or the birth outcome. The goal is to practice the known traditions that provide relief and healing and allow new mothers to claim their heralded new status.

Special Note: Losing a Baby

If you have experienced the loss of a baby, whether from an early miscarriage, a late miscarriage, or a stillbirth, you still deserve support and to honor the African American postpartum traditions. Your womb carried a life, and you birthed a baby. You have the same physiological needs and a more intense emotional need because you don't have your baby to hold and care for. I am so sorry for your loss.

I have seen mothers who had late miscarriages return to work within two days, believing that they did not deserve or need postpartum care. Many of them became ill with uterine infections, acute backaches, depression, and general unease.[6] You deserve to be cared for and loved, regardless of your birth outcome. Please accept the care as you grieve.

CELEBRATE THE POWER OF MOTHERHOOD

Before colonization, African women were held in high esteem because of their leadership and ability to birth and nurture new life, the most important aspect of family/village survival. Reclaiming this position of mother will give you a sense of being well loved and highly respected. Our traditions and rituals create balance in the body and resolve conflict within the mind as we navigate the humbling journey of transformation and growth. Motherhood is a sacred passage. Our traditions maintain trust in the community and restore the natural order of a mother having time and space to heal as she watches her baby acclimate and grow. Let us take what we have fetched from the past and use it to thrive as mothers.

PART TWO

Mother and Newborn Care from Africa: The Principles of African American Postpartum Traditions

CHAPTER 3

Honored and Prayed Over

May you be honored during your postpartum period. Fussed and hovered over. May you have family and community to put a pillow under your head, prop your feet up, draw you a bath, bring you warm food, and hold your baby so you can sleep. May you be sung to and prayed over. May you feel spiritually and emotionally cared for and connected to a greater purpose. Know that you are lovingly held by your Creator, protected and held by an infinite power. People are rooting for you; you are not alone. They are pouring energy into your healing and growth.

Dear Creator, bless this mother from worry. Give her strength in body, abundant breastmilk with easy breastfeeding, and bless her baby to be a help to their family and society. God, bless the mother with strong Motherwit so she can know the best way to help herself, her baby, and all of her household.

HONOR AND PRAYER ARE IMPORTANT ASPECTS OF SOCIAL SUPPORT, a fundamental principle for good postpartum care. It shows the new mother that she is loved, cared for, and held in high esteem. Through honor and prayer, we manifest a form of healing that is multidimensional and spiritual, directly connected to

African knowledge. For us, spirituality is our lineage, and healing enters through the heart. We were born from ancestors who prayed for our liberation from enslavement, relief from suffering, and healing back to wholeness. We continue their legacy when we honor and pray for ourselves and one another as mothers.

The Three Essences of Honored and Prayed Over
1. The mind carries emotions.
2. The body carries the burden from birth.
3. The soul connects to the spiritual or the supernatural.

When a mother has returned to the physical after birth, we say a simple prayer: "Thank God, she made it." We recognize that while birth is natural and most births are problem-free, some mothers will not return from it. That is why prayers, along with stellar health care, remain an integral part of postpartum care. When I brought a problem to my grandma, she would say, "Well, did you pray?" Praying for and over a new mother is customary as a form of protection. New mothers need prayers to help them transition back to the nonpregnant state and into motherhood.

Honoring the mother is a postpartum practice that exceeds general care. We treat the mother as nobility, honor her with honesty and integrity, and show her respect and admiration. Honoring the mother can take many forms, but it is best when it shows up through daily consistent interactions that support her ongoing wellness, like providing nourishing meals, giving her daily back rubs, gifting her fresh flowers and maintaining them for her, praising her and validating her ability to be physically healed from birth, complimenting her mothering and postpartum vitality, and offering a sympathetic ear to her daily challenges as a mother. Every honoring gesture helps the mother feel seen and cared for.

As soon as I walk in the door to my postpartum mothers' homes, I pray. I ask the Creator to let me know what needs to be done, and I set my intention: *Let me be a light to her; let me help her feel the best she can. If she isn't telling me something I need to know, give me the intuition I need to support her.*

Our ancestral healing practices are holistic, tending to the mind, body, and soul to attain positive postpartum healing. The elders would say, "Before you fix your body, you need to fix your mind," "You need to pray that sickness out of you," and "There is something wrong; I can feel it in my spirit." While we have been denied this spiritual art for various reasons, we still remember it in our DNA, and our souls feel happy and fulfilled when a new mother is honored properly. Prayer and honor has a way of reminding Black mothers to tap into their faith to keep their emotions positive and reduce postpartum depression.[1]

Honoring and praying over postpartum mothers supersedes all physical support, like nutrition, heat, herbs, and more. It must come first. If you are the mother, your task is to learn to let others honor you. If you are a family member, friend, or community member of a new mother, your job is to understand the sacred art of celebrating and praying over her and removing any guilt that will prevent her from resting.

Black Women, Rest

We built America on the back of our motherhood. Resting during postpartum is our culture, relaxing is our birthright, and self-care is our human right. It is time we take back what we have been denied for decades, and that is the right to rest and recuperate after birth and nurture our new baby.

African Art Honors the Mother

In Mother Africa, the fertile land where life began and motherhood is honored, mothers are memorialized through art, the most ancient and powerful form of communication. This can be found in most African cultures, especially among the Khemit, Dogon, and Bantu people. These cultures believed in the Creator and honored the natural order of the universe. Honoring the Creator through inherent respect, service, and love for those in need, like the vulnerable, the sick, and mothers, is a crucial aspect of compassion in ancient African civilizations. These are eternal testimonials showing the honor that dynasties and empires bestowed on the mother as a life giver and a direct communicator with the life force of God.

African artifacts show reverence for the mother through kinship, community, and her high position in the societal order of her people. Mother statues are often placed in sacred locations to cultivate peace and protect the children and the future. Wood carvings and bronze, iron, and gold sculptures frequently depict pregnant women and breastfeeding mothers with elongated breasts. The imagery also includes women holding children's hands, babies wrapped on their backs, and mothers walking with small children.

As African Americans, we must celebrate the diversity of African art that rekindles our shared sense of humanity, which begins with the eternally powerful image of a mother and her baby. Honoring motherhood is in our DNA. It's our healing culture and our gratitude for the one who carried us and brought us into the physical world.

WHAT IT MEANS TO BE HONORED

Honor in African American culture is multifaceted. It includes how you speak to and address the new mother and the tone you use when speaking in her presence. It was said that the Granny Midwives spoke lovingly and with empathy and babied the mother when talking with her. They would approach her with endearment, a positive attitude, and a slow, matter-of-fact, slightly authoritative style. Today, we want to do the same while still allowing the mother to have her say on what she wants. This approach shows respect and reverence.

We measure how well we are honoring the postpartum mother based on her response, which she can verbalize or show with her body language. On the flip side, as a new mother, when you are being honored, you should feel calm, in control of your surroundings, and emotionally cared for. Many attribute these good feelings to the release of oxytocin, the love hormone, which is often released when you feel safe, listened to, respected, encouraged, and held in high esteem.

We honor the mother with positive talk about how brave and special she is, and she is repeatedly reminded of sacred texts, history, evidence-based research, and stories from other mothers who can share their postpartum experiences. I have found that mothers love to hear how motherhood was honored in different African tribes and how this looked for African Americans in the twentieth century. It is an honor to know that people are proud of you, happy for you, rooting for you, and pouring energy into your healing and growth as a mother.

NOT-SO-NEW NEW MOMS

Regardless of how many babies you have birthed, you are a new mother each time you give birth, and you have the same postpartum needs, sometimes even more. Many experienced mothers receive less postpartum support with each child they birth because society believes that they know what they are doing and can be more independent. At the same time, mothers who already have one or more children sometimes decline postpartum support because they don't think they need the help or, worse, they don't think they have the time to receive help. This is far from the truth. All postpartum mothers need physical and emotional support after the birth of their baby, whether it's their first or their fifth. The mother should feel safe to ask questions and get her needs met. Let's listen to a Black woman when she speaks; she knows exactly what she needs.

Serving the mother in all its forms is another way of honoring her. Serving can look like bringing her meals and removing the plates when she is finished; sincerely asking if there is anything else that can be done to help her get more comfortable in mind, body, and spirit; spontaneously laying another blanket over her because it feels drafty; or cracking a window because it feels stuffy or even smelly in the room. I honor a new mother by giving her a warm, loving hug when I enter her room and when I leave for the day, unless she is asleep, in which case, I simply check on her. When I walk into the mother's space and see an empty glass, I honor her by filling it back up because a postpartum mother must stay hydrated. I also honor her with my words by telling her that she looks beautiful, she's doing a great job, she is blessed and amazing, and she deserves to be treated like a queen.

Being honored builds confidence, and that can be a lifesaver for Black women who are typically not honored or adequately cared for in the Western medical healthcare system or mainstream society. The stress that comes with not being heard can contribute to postpartum depression, maternal illness, and even death.[2] According to the research, Black women's concerns and needs going unaddressed is a major contributing factor to the disproportionate rate of Black maternal mortality in the US healthcare system. Our traditions can help eradicate these injustices by giving mothers their rightful powerful positions to advocate for themselves.

HONORING YOURSELF AND YOUR MOTHERWIT

The first forty-two days after birth are a vulnerable time because your body is beginning to heal and there may be a lot of emotions, both good and bad. There may be times when you feel unsure of your mothering skills and what to expect in the postpartum period, you experience physical discomforts, you have breastfeeding challenges, or you have a hard time soothing your infant. These challenges are typical, but can make you doubt your capabilities. This is the time to own your Motherwit. Know that you know how to help your baby. The key is to listen to and honor your mothering voice and body. Act how you feel is best, and gather the information you need from this book. You can always call your healthcare provider if you feel at a complete loss.

You know if you feel tired, achy, or overwhelmed. You can honor yourself during this time by responding to your feelings and bodily sensations. If you are tired, rest. If your body aches, use your heating pad, take a very warm shower, or get a massage. Honoring yourself validates that you are capable and builds confidence. With or without support, you are honorable. Enjoy this time of reflection with your baby.

HONORING THE BABY

I always tell new mothers, "Honor your baby as you honor yourself, and keep your baby close to you." Babies have personalities, and some need much attention, which can be tiring for a new mother. One way to support and honor yourself and your baby is to learn how to safely share a bed, which allows you to respond quickly when your baby cries, lessening their distress and reducing your fatigue because you don't have to keep getting out of bed to care for them. To soothe your baby, you can pick them up with love and confidence and/or use your breast as a pacifier, which also helps reduce your chances of hemorrhaging in the first forty-two days after birth. If your baby keeps crying after using these methods, undress them down to their diaper and do continuous skin-to-skin contact.

There is a saying that babies don't cry in Africa. This is because in many African cultures, breastfeeding is on demand, everyone immediately picks up a crying baby, and family members keep new babies close to them with baby-wearing, either in the front or the back. Don't listen to people who say that quickly attending to your baby's needs is spoiling them. Babies are a gift and a blessing. You cannot spoil them; you can only love them. The concept of "spoiling a baby" is a direct result of post-traumatic slave syndrome that our ancestors experienced, which was based on the violence of being separated from their children during slavery. It is our job now to reclaim our traditional and spiritual parenting methods of keeping our babies close, showering them with love and care, and nurturing them into confident individuals. They lived inside you for a long time, so it only makes sense that they feel safer and better when they are near you. What a blessing!

Tips for Honoring the Baby

- Hold your baby skin to skin.
- Sing and talk to your baby.
- Keep your baby clean and warm.
- Breastfeed on demand.
- Let your breast be a pacifier.
- Burp your baby after meals.
- Bed-share safely.
- Respond immediately to your baby's cries.
- Trust your Motherwit.
- Remember that newborns cannot be spoiled.
- Love and enjoy your baby.
- Smell and kiss your baby throughout the day.
- Let people you trust hold your baby.
- Don't engage with phones and computer screens when holding your baby.

HOW TO HONOR THE MOTHER

I didn't have family or communal support when my first baby was born because my mother had passed and my sisters and friends did not know what they should be doing. I had a good husband, but he went to work the day after I gave birth. So, I was home alone with my baby from the start of our lives together. The house was quiet, with no visitors and minimal calls. I didn't feel honored or celebrated, but I was content and happy with my baby, fed myself easy foods, rested on the couch the majority of the day, and nursed my baby when he cried. When my husband came home after work, he would cook and we would eat together. As a result, I had a wonderful recuperation and a happy baby.

With that said, it's ideal that you, your baby, and your partner are well honored by your community, and this—as you'll learn in the coming pages—can come in many forms. Be innovative in asking others to honor you properly and find creative ways to honor yourself in the process.

How You Can Honor Yourself

- List your accomplishments in real time.
- Trust yourself, your body, and your Motherwit.
- Eat often. Say yes if food is offered.
- Keep yourself warm.
- Rest and enjoy your baby; it is a part of our culture to do this!

General Ways to Honor Mama

- List her accomplishments in real time to uplift her.
- Accept her perspective on how she wants to heal and nurture her baby.

- Show her value and give her respect, care, and a sense of empowerment.
- Accompany her when she moves about, assist her in sitting and getting up, and elevate her feet.
- Bring her beverages and savory snacks.
- Keep her warm.
- Pay for a postpartum doula to visit daily for the first six weeks.
- Send a daily positive text.
- Stop by to help with household tasks, like cooking, cleaning, or laundry.

Every honoring gesture helps the mother feel seen and cared about and prevents exhaustion, which can greatly reduce her chances of developing postpartum depression.[3]

Asking and Receiving Questions

A new mother, particularly a first-time mother, will likely have a lot of questions. When I make a home visit as a midwife, I like to assure the mother that all her questions are important and that there are no stupid ones. I tell her she can always call or text me as questions arise. This simple practice of giving the mother confidence to ask questions can help her feel comfortable enough to advocate for herself and her baby in the outside world, especially in medical environments.

In many African traditions, women's voices are respected, which we can see has been maintained in our culture with our grandmother's implied authority and the many Black female leaders throughout history that we look up to. When we encourage new mothers to ask questions and voice their concerns, we are giving their voices back, reclaiming our own, and ensuring that the women in our lives feel heard and understood. This is so important for two reasons: One, worry and anxiety can affect breastmilk supply, and two, Black women have historically suffered greatly from preventable illnesses by not being listened to. When our community encourages equal and open dialogue, it expels the myths that motherhood is a burden and models for the next generation how we traditionally navigate and honor motherhood.

CELEBRATE YOUR BEAUTY

So many women have bought into the myth that their bodies should be like they were before they had a baby. This leads many women to say things, like "How soon can I get my body back? I hate my body. What's going to happen to my breasts if I breastfeed my baby?" In an effort to get their bodies to "snap back," new mothers are jogging with babies in strollers as soon as they can, but this can have adverse effects on health and postpartum recovery. Science says that a certain amount of fat is needed to maintain a healthy level of postpartum hormones for breastfeeding, brain health, and stress management.[4]

On top of this, Black women have the added impact of melanin, which darkens the stomach, breasts, and sometimes even the face during pregnancy.[5] I'm here to let you know that melanin is part of the beauty of motherhood, and embracing this can help you better understand your identity as a Black woman and break away from the harmful stereotypes of motherhood. This is why African American postpartum traditions recognize the increased melanin that results from pregnancy hormones and welcome it as both natural and beautiful. The postpartum body is stunning, with its dark linea nigra on the belly, its deep silver stretch marks that develop over the uterus, and its chocolate areolas and large nipples that command your baby's, and partner's, attention. All women will not develop all of these traits, but we can see them as beautiful because they are all cultural. I like to say that the beautiful stretch marks on dark skin are like the reflection of the moon's light upon the rippling ocean waves on a dark night.

Your postpartum body is beautiful. Define your own beauty standards. You are beautiful; you always were. Love yourself, and do not compare yourself to others.

Beautifying Rituals

When a mother is fussed over and beautified, she feels better emotionally, which makes her feel better about herself and caring for her baby. Here are a few beautifying rituals you can do to honor the new mother:

- Help her with daily hygiene, like showering and bathing.
- Do her hair, oil her scalp, and wrap it all in a silk or satin scarf (no need for long hair-care regimens, as this can tire mama out).
- Oil her skin with relaxing African postpartum healing oils, like coconut, sesame, frankincense, or jasmine.
- Massage warmed henna paste on her nails, in the center of her hands, or on the bottom of her feet as decoration.
- Put on blessed jewelry, like a necklace, after her shower.
- Dress her in a beautiful gown or African Bubu dress for easy breastfeeding.
- Wrap her belly with scented African cloth or indigo blue cloth (African fabric has a healing vibration).

SACRED PRAYER

Prayer is what got us through the Middle Passage, enslavement, Jim Crow, and the racism that continues for Black people in the

United States today. Spirituality and prayer are part of the richness and beauty of the Black American tradition that enslaved Africans brought with them to America.[6] This spiritual medicine has never ended; it is expressed by kneeling in front of a chair or bed, holding hands, calling on the Creator or "getting the spirit," and being prayed over. Granny Midwives always included spirituality with root medicines when they taught families how to care for new mothers.[7] (I'll share more about herbal medicines in chapter 7.)

Prayer was very intentional and organized for early African American midwives. Families and individuals gathered by appointment to pray for the new mother and baby. Part of the postpartum ritual was sitting in a circle outside the mother's bedroom and saying her name aloud in the prayer.[8] Other methods included sending protection by praying in the room where the mother slept or praying over her while she laid in bed. When we pray with or for the mother, we strengthen the spiritual connection between her and her baby, the community, and the higher power. Prayer can be just between you and mama; it can be a call-and-response, with the response being a simple "Amen" or "Ashe"; or you can make it your own. You could form a healing circle around the mother and anoint her with blessed oils and flora water, or you could lay your hands over her and send her positive energy.

Praying as a new mother or over a new mother greatly impacts postpartum recovery because it provides hope and brings spiritual healing from the highest source of life, the Creator. Prayer empowers you to tap into something bigger than yourself and know that you can affect your healing and face challenges because you have a connection to a higher power that lives both within and outside you.

Praying and being prayed over is a natural and organic ritual for the postpartum mother, her baby, and her family. Even if you're not used to being prayed over as a new mother, you probably have a natural desire to have good wishes given to you and to feel held by your community's support. Prayer allows us to do something practical to help ourselves. It gives us a way to articulate our soul-deep concerns and needs and receive solutions. The gift of prayer is available to all postpartum mothers, regardless of their age, religion, location, or marital status.

Call-and-Response Prayer

In its simplest form, praying over a postpartum mother includes a call-and-response format—you call out and the mother answers back. Call-and-response is a spiritual form of communication that links back to Africa and continues today. The person initiating the prayer asks for a response from the listeners, and their response is an acknowledgment that everyone is in agreement with the prayer and that they are adding their personal power to it.

An example of a call-and-response prayer is: "Dear God, we pray that you bless this new mother with health and healing and that she has joy in motherhood and peace when sleeping. We pray that all her needs—physically, mentally, and emotionally—be met. We pray that her baby is healthy and happy. We thank you, God, for safely bringing her and her baby through the birth journey. Bless her." Then, the person leading the prayer will say, "Can I get an Amen?" and everyone involved will respond with "Amen." The response can also be anything that the listener feels moved by their spirit to say or do, perhaps a hum, a snap, a clap, or other interjections, like "Hallelujah," "Praise God," or "Allahu Akbar (God is great)."

I love being involved in the call-and-response prayer ritual. It can become very rhythmic, and it is a form of healing that includes everyone's positive vibrations and good energy. When I get to respond to a prayer, I feel complete because my energy is now part of the collective.

PRAYER PRACTICES

The ways I pray over the mother are the culmination of what has been passed down in my family and what I have learned from other Black midwives and healers. You can and should let your practices emerge from your family and community traditions first. I do some form of prayer at every visit. Some are verbal, some are silent, but they all work with good intentions. The honor comes from giving the mother my full attention so she knows she is the most important person in the room.

In my typical prayer ritual, I like to sit alone with a new mother and pray over her. These prayers are always organic and from my heart. To begin, I wash my hands and pray over them in private, then I anoint her hands in a bowl of warm water, pull up a chair beside her bed, take both of her hands in mine, and say, "Let's pray." Then, I lead the prayer: "Dear God, bless this new mother, answer all her needs, those seen and unseen, and give her gratitude, hope, and wisdom to care for herself and her newborn."

Or I may do a longer prayer, such as:

Bless this mother with a quick and complete recuperation, protecting her from all postpartum illnesses of body and mind. May all her internal parts be healed, and may only good surround her and all negativities stay far removed from her. I pray she will be joyful and have a healthy and thriving infant, with a partner full of understanding and love for the new mother.

I like my prayers to acknowledge the mother's rite of passage and ask for her to cross it safely and securely. I like to invite healing and protection and ignite the family's gratitude and spiritual strength in bringing solace to the mother and remembrance of God. Most mothers tell me they feel better during and after the prayer, and I feel better too for making the prayer on her behalf. It is an energy exchange—a ritual, a beautiful moment of reflection and faith.

When leaving her home, I say out loud, "God bless and protect this home and give peace to those who reside here."

Honoring Mama with Prayer

Your prayers are meant to restore good health to the mother and keep the new baby strong and healthy as well. Think of these prayers as a form of encouragement as your family walks the postpartum journey day by day. The prayer holds the postpartum mother to the tradition of allowing herself to be taken care of, asking for and expecting help, and setting boundaries from the outside world to honor the rituals of the lying-in period. Prayer is personal for each individual; however, there are some ways you can pray for the postpartum mama:

- Talk to God.
- Be specific with your prayer.

- Believe that your prayer will be answered.
- Be thankful and anxious for nothing.
- Keep the faith.

Set Your Intentions

- Ask for protection from illness and negative energy.
- Pray that she will be a successful mother and can manage normal postpartum challenges, both emotional and physical.
- Show gratitude to the Creator for the mother and baby's life.
- Call upon all that is sacred to help the new mother and her baby find harmony within and be strong. Ask that they not fall ill so they can enter society with strength when the postpartum period is completed.
- Remember your ancestors and call their names because they are still family.

When you pray with intention and earnestness, you're fostering a sense of unity and harmony within your community. Your prayers are a vigil that keeps the community engaged, even if people cannot show up physically. You can certainly hold prayer over Zoom or on the phone with the new mother present.

Prayer can come in many modes: silent, verbal, weeping, long, short, planned or spontaneous, collective or individual. You can write down your prayer and include chants and words of affirmation. You can put pages of Holy Scripture or poems under the new mother's mattress or leave a spiritual book in her bedroom. Singing hymns, spirituals, songs, and chants is also a form of prayer that bestows blessings and protection on the new mother and her newborn. Some families even call in their pastor, imam, or spiritual leader to make prayer in the mother's home, or they send a request to their faith congregation to announce the birth and ask for a collective prayer for the health of the baby and mother.

WHEN YOU HONOR THE MOTHER, YOU HONOR ALL MOTHERS AND THE ANCESTORS

Giving birth deserves honor. It is not a negative. It is positive. Yet the journey of postpartum recovery is a mixed experience of physical and emotional changes and discomfort as the body, mind, and spirit heal. Major organs must return to their original size and place in the body. Honor and prayer is how we generate the positive energy needed for the mother's health, strength, and well-being. When we honor and pray over the new mother, we participate in age-old traditions, with roots in ancient Africa, to celebrate the uniqueness of the female experience. We emotionally and spiritually claim that the mother is the most special and the most beautiful and that she deserves all the love and support because she did the hard work of bringing forth new life. We affirm the sacredness of her life. We show we are invested in her emotional and spiritual health and healing. As a community and a family, we assert that she matters to us. We create safety for her. When we pray over the mother, we develop a foundation of love and compassion that resonates beyond the boundaries of time and space and upholds our ancestral traditions of mothering.

CHAPTER 4

Warmed

Dear new mother,
Congratulations! You opened yourself both spiritually and phys-
ically to birth your baby into the world, and now, it is time to
retreat to the warm love between you and your baby. You are
warm, you are loved, and you are wrapped in the healing rays
of motherhood. May you absorb the healing heat from every area
of your life and feel revived, in harmony, and at peace. Imagine
yourself wrapped in Grandma's heated quilt, which has messages
for you: Don't worry about anything. Trust that you know what
to do for you and your baby. In your warmth, you will find your
way to health, happiness, and power. Follow the warm path, and
it will lead you to wellness. I love you.

MY SECOND BABY, A DAUGHTER, WAS BORN ON SEPTEMBER 11, AND
I remember feeling her cool and damp body when she was
placed on my bare skin. She was so soft. I remember rubbing my
hands over her smooth body to warm her up. It was such a beautiful time. Once my midwife covered us both with a blanket, heat
generated between us, and we both became the perfect temperature for each other. Creating warmth and keeping her warm in the

first hours after her birth was instinctive; I kept gently rubbing my inner arm over various parts of her to make sure she stayed warm.

Heat and warmth are fundamental to postpartum healing, and can come from a variety of sources like the sun, blankets, heated stones, and warm sand. The Granny Midwife's main priority was keeping the new mother and newborn warm. She knew that warmth creates feelings of comfort and emotional balance, and she also wanted to ensure that the new mother stayed healthy enough to make it through the first forty days of the postpartum period, when most maternal deaths occur.[1] The midwife would put a scarf on the mother's head, blankets over her body, and keep the fireplace going to keep the postpartum room warm. The Granny Midwife also believed that warmth could be used as a medical therapy for healing.

She had it right. Research has confirmed that heat increases the extensibility of collagen tissues, decreases joint stiffness, reduces pain and inflammation, relieves muscle spasms, aids in the post-acute phase of healing, and increases blood flow to injured areas.[2] A study using warmed blankets on elders in residential care facilities showed a significant decrease in pain level, agitation, physical complaints, and the severity of complaints.[3] Likewise, in postpartum contexts, warmed blankets reduce chills and bring comfort to new mothers. Staying warm after birth is essential to maintain a healthy immune system, especially in cold weather and drafty environments.[4]

You should be warmed immediately after the birth of your baby, so tell your birth assistants and family members and add it to your birth plan. Hospital rooms are especially cold, so you want to make sure that your nurse changes you into a dry gown and puts a dry sheet under you and a warmed blanket over you and the baby right away. You'll also want to wear slippers. This will begin postpartum healing. Warmth is like being wrapped in the cocoon of the womb or being embraced by the warm arms of your mother or loved ones. During the postpartum period, there will be times when it will be difficult to comfort your crying baby, you'll be faced with different emotional demands, and you'll experience postpartum discomforts, like engorged breasts. This is the perfect time to apply heat and warmth to the areas that are aching or retreat under a warm blanket with or without your baby to settle your mind. Applying heat to the body will help you relax, which can help you cope better with the situation in front of you.

When I think of being warm, so many good memories come to mind, like tightly hugging a loved one, lying under a cozy blanket or in the sun, sipping my favorite hot beverage in my favorite house robe, eating a hot soup or a spicy meal, sitting in front of the fireplace, or having a warm massage.

WARMTH IS MEDICINE

Growing up, I was taught the importance of staying warm and avoiding the cold. Heat is integrated into every aspect of Black culture, from hot baths to spicy food. We woke up to piping hot grits, hot rice cereal, hot eggs, and meat, accompanied with hot drinks like herbal teas. During my childhood, parents often insisted that their children keep warm indoors and out. The elders believed that you lost most of your body heat through the top of your head and the bottom of your feet, so as children, we were told to keep our heads and feet covered on chilly days and, when ill, to keep these areas covered to heal faster by preventing the healing warmth from escaping our body. When indoors, it was the culture to keep socks or slippers on our feet when walking on cold surfaces. Elders would say, "Put something on," even if you were fully dressed. They meant that you should put on a sweater or long-sleeved clothes; otherwise, it was believed that you would catch a cold.

Chilly weather or being cold was associated with an array of health problems for all age groups: Babies got gripe or colic, new mothers got sick from getting cold in their wombs, and elders suffered from joint pain in cold temperatures. Our healing remedies were always about heat. If you were sick, the prescription was to lay under quilts or wool blankets with a hot water bottle, Bengay, and hot tea. The goal was to sweat it out—"it" being the illness or toxins. This all comes from the African American belief in thermal healing. Wearing a hat outdoors in the winter was nonnegotiable. Even if your coat had a hood, your mother or grandmother likely still made you wear a hat under it to prevent the cold from getting in your ears, which was believed to cause earaches. There are even some records of Granny Midwives putting cotton in the ears of new mothers for that very reason: to prevent the cold from getting into her body and causing disease.

The Granny Midwives believed that birth made the inside of the body cold because internal heat was lost with the opening of the womb. It was believed that if left open and exposed to cold, the mother would feel weak, which could lead to postpartum illnesses and discomfort. When a postpartum mother's body is left open, she is more susceptible to sickness, such as arthritis in her joints and bones and a more difficult menopause experience later in life. Granny Midwives knew what science has confirmed: Increased exposure to cold lowers the immune system. It makes the body use more energy, increasing the need for more calories to keep the internal temperature at 98.6°F, or 37°C. She knew from the traditional healers that heat helps the body heal and relieves the soreness that comes from birthing by increasing blood circulation and bringing oxygen to injured areas.

Historically, in the South, the mother's family would warm the postpartum room by sealing the windows and keeping the fireplace burning daily during the first forty-two days. The father and other people in the community would help by supplying wood. The tradition was that the ashes from the fireplace could not be swept up until the lying-in period was over. Putting hot bricks under the bed was also an effective practice, as well as placing wool blankets or quilts on mama. Scarves were often tied on the mother's head, and her feet were covered with socks. A new mother should never allow her feet to touch a cold floor.

Granny Midwives used various methods to create internal and environmental heat. For external warming methods, they would heat a kettle of water and create warm compresses out of cloth folded in fourths and soaked in hot water. They would then apply these to any aching areas, like the breasts, the abdomen, the upper and lower back, and the vulva. They also wrapped heated stones in cloth and put them at the foot of the bed to trap heat under the blankets. These traditions continue today with the use of hot water bottles, heated rice socks, electrical heating pads or warming blankets, and space heaters.

Many pregnant women enter their labor with lower back aches, pelvic pain, breast tenderness, nausea, headaches, leg cramps, and sore arches. These are similar to postpartum discomforts, which are then compounded with new physical and emotional symptoms that are the result of the actual birth, like vulva pain. With the birth of the baby, there is normal pressure on the anal region, which can lead to hemorrhoids and tailbone pain. Applying heat to these sore areas helps reduce discomfort and increase circulation, aiding the recuperation process. Other postpartum discomforts that benefit from heat and warmth are pain from a cesarean incision, involution pain, breast engorgement, sore or cracked nipples, upper to mid-back pain from an epidural injection site, and aching legs from being held while pushing. Heat and warmth bring circulation to all these areas, providing immediate comfort in some cases and comfort in a few days to weeks in others.

When you stay warm, you are more likely to feel relaxed, have a deeper sleep, and wake up feeling refreshed. This is important because we manage pain better when we are well-rested. The heat will also help your muscles relax, eliminating the tension that may have resulted from labor or positioning during your pushing stage.

The Advantages of Thermotherapy

- **Increasing blood flow:** Heat dilates blood vessels, allowing more oxygen and nutrients to reach the muscles and promoting relaxation.
- **Improving flexibility:** Warm muscles are more pliable, which can reduce stiffness and improve range of motion.
- **Easing pain:** Heat stimulates sensory receptors in the skin, which can reduce the perception of pain in the area.
- **Soothing stress:** The comfort of warmth can help calm the nervous system, further relaxing tense muscles.[5]

Practical Warming Methods

- Warming methods include postpartum baths, hot showers, heating pads, hot compresses, and massages with warm oils (such as mustard seed oil, clove oil, olive oil, warm shea butter, or coconut oil).
- There are also simple warming acts, like keeping mama's feet covered with socks while in the bed, wearing slippers when walking on cold surfaces, and wearing a robe in cool or cold environments.

- Vaginal steaming is another comforting, warming postpartum tradition. As a new mother, you can sit on a chair or stool with a large pot full of boiled rosemary underneath. Once you are sitting on the chair over the steam pot, you can then wrap yourself in blankets or towels from head to toe to trap the steam inside. The steam will warm and heal your vulva and pelvic region. After steaming or a postpartum bath, apply warm oil on your abdomen, and if it feels good, ask your support person to wrap your stomach to hold warmth in the uterus and pelvic areas.
- Use your Motherwit to think about how to keep yourself warm. Make sure you don't sit on cold surfaces like metal folding chairs; wooden kitchen chairs; stone, tiled, or iron benches; or cold steps. Put a folded blanket, quilt, or cotton pillow on all cold surfaces before sitting on them. Preferably, you should sit on upholstered chairs and avoid leather car seats until the car has been warmed up or the built-in seat warmers have kicked in. If you give birth during the summer, when most surfaces are warmed by the sun, it can feel great to sit on them, but be careful that the surfaces are not dangerously hot.
- I remember one bright Alabama day in December when I left my grandmother's porch to sit on the brick steps to get direct sunlight. I was holding my six-month-old son and enjoying the warmth and the view of the beautiful field in front of her house. When my grandmother saw me sitting on the cold brick steps, she told me to get up and never sit on a cold surface or I would "get cold in my womb," and it would create a difficult menopause. I was

twenty-one years old when she told me this, and I have never sat on a cold surface since.

- Along with the physical warming traditions, there are warm foods that will help you gain strength in your immediate postpartum period. Warming foods help boost metabolism and increase the heart rate, which improves alertness and energy—essential benefits to a new mother. The other benefit is that warming foods often have higher calories and more nutrients to support the female body, and they help widen the blood vessels, which improves the oxygen and nutrient flow through the body.[6] Also you are more likely to enjoy the taste and smell of warm foods.

- The first step is to eat a warm protein soup or broth immediately after birth, even as you are breastfeeding. Soups that are heavily seasoned with hot spices, like peppers, curry, garlic, chilies, cloves, nutmeg, onions, and cayenne, and are left to simmer on the stove or in the Crock-Pot will warm your insides and help with digestion and elimination. When I help postpartum moms, I make them a hot curry chicken coconut soup with finely chopped greens and chicken parts, including chicken livers, which are added for more iron. At home births, soup is sometimes fed to the mother even before the placenta is expelled.

- Offer caffeine-free warming teas, like mint, cinnamon, lemon, cayenne and ginger, turmeric with black peppercorn, raspberry, and clove teas, sweetened for taste with honey. All warm herbal teas are good, but spicier teas create heat in the stomach, which help aid digestion.

- Other warming liquids include hot water with lemon and honey, warm milk and honey, and warmed apple juice.

Like the Granny Midwife, it's important that you are creative in creating warmth. For example, you can move your bed away from any windows, cover windows with plastic and add heavy curtains, add space heaters to your room, and keep extra blankets, socks, hair bonnets, and scarves on hand to facilitate warmth.

The warming should begin in the hospital as well. I tell mothers in the hospital to step right into their slippers when getting out of bed. Most mothers complain about how cold they are during their hospital stay, so it's vital that warming rituals are practiced right away and continued at home.

The body's transition to its nonpregnant state should be supported with traditional warming practices. Ask your support people to help you stay warm by bringing hot water bottles wrapped in a towel or a heated rice sock, running a hot bath, or even getting you a cup of hot tea. Have someone put hot compresses on your lower back, bring your slippers, or put nonslip socks on your feet. Helping to keep a new mother warm is easy and makes a big difference in a positive postpartum recuperation.

CLOSING THE BODY

Through birth, you become open and vulnerable as the cervix and birth canal widen for the baby to enter the world. Once the baby is born, the body must be closed. Get a hot water bottle, wrap it in a towel, and put it on your lower abdomen; eat one of the recipes from this book; and after you have completed your forty-two-day lying-in period, end with a ritual of walking clockwise three times around the outside of your house or apartment building (or inside if cold), holding a small cup of water and your child. Drink the water when you reach the front of your house on the third circle. This is a Granny Midwife tradition that confirms you can reenter society. But by all means continue to take it slow for the first year.

WARMING PRACTICES IMMEDIATELY AFTER BIRTH

The most fundamental warming ritual for baby and mama is skin-to-skin contact immediately after birth or as soon as possible after birth. Your baby will be placed on your bare skin to help you bond and create heat. Once the baby is warm, they'll return the heat to you. I have heard many mothers say, "My baby is so hot." This means that their baby is now able to regulate its own body temperature. While the mom is bonding with the baby, someone can feed the mother a hot soup or tea, which gets her circulation moving and begins the healing warming period. We never give cold food or drinks because it reduces oxygen flow to the injured body and delays healing.

After birth, I also apply a very warm washcloth to the vaginal area. And I often do this during the pushing phase as well. I've been catching babies for forty years, and I always use this warmth practice. Every mother who I warmed with hot water compresses said it helped them push more efficiently, and mothers who had previous births without this tradition often commented, "I needed this with my other babies." It can be done at home or in the hospital; in fact a version of this has become common practice during and after hospital births, so make sure you talk to your providers about it.

For my home birth compresses, I usually stew comfrey and rosemary together on the stove. Comfrey aids in cell regeneration, and rosemary serves as an antiseptic. Once the pushing begins, I turn the stove to low heat, strain the tea into a bowl, and keep it nearby with three white cotton facecloths. Immediately after birth and before the placenta is expelled, I put a warm cloth on the vulva for comfort. This is considered a wet-heat application. After the placenta is expelled, I put a clean dry sheet under mom, and if she has gotten wet from her ruptured membranes, blood, or sweat, I help her into warm, clean, dry clothes and continue applying warm compresses to her vulva. I then put a blanket over her shoulders or her body, and make sure the new baby is covered and warmed as well.

There are also dry-heat applications. If the house is drafty, consider putting a hat on the baby's head and a scarf on mom's. Use extra blankets, hot water bottles, or heating pads on the bed or her aching body parts. Make sure the new mother has socks on her feet. Bringing warmth to the uterus with dry-heat methods helps some mothers deal with the pain that comes with the shrinking of the uterus.

New mothers need to feel warmed up immediately after birth to ignite the internal postpartum healing process and feel loved, cared for, and safe.

WARMING YOUR NEWBORN

Just as it's healing to warm the mother, warming the newborn is considered essential infant care in the African American postpartum tradition. With all seven of my babies, I followed the tradition of covering their heads and feet and wrapping them in cotton receiving blankets when taking them outside the home. For my five babies who were born in the summer, I covered their heads and feet with summer fabrics, and for my two November babies, I used warmer materials.

Hospitals have a similar practice of immediately putting a hat on the newborn to prevent them from losing body heat from the largest surface of their body, which is their head. The medical goal is to warm the baby back to 98.6°F, as their temperature drops when they leave the warmth of the womb and enter the cold outside world. This is why skin to skin is excellent for maintaining warmth for the newborn.

Additionally, in African American postpartum tradition, babies are typically not taken outside the home for the first six weeks, except for pediatric appointments. Stemming from several African traditions, babies were also kept away from nonfamily members and public places for spiritual and physical protection.[7] When you do go out with your baby, dress them how you dress yourself, meaning if you wear socks and shoes in cold weather, so should your baby. Too often, I see babies out in cold weather without socks, shoes, a hat, or a blanket, but the parent is dressed appropriately. At the same time, medicine advises not to overdress babies because it can contribute to overheating. Overdressing babies in summer or in a hot house can cause this. The signs of overheating are skin that is hot to the touch, a red or flushed face, damp skin around the neck or forehead, rapid breathing, lethargy, irritability, or fussiness. To stop overheating, unwrap the baby, take off their hat and socks, and move them to a cooler area in the shade or where there is a natural breeze. You could also breastfeed them or give them a few teaspoons of cool spring water.

I experienced overheating with my firstborn. I was breastfeeding him in public under a blanket for modesty. When he stopped nursing, I took him from under the blanket. He was so red and wet with perspiration that I panicked. I immediately began to undress him to bring his temperature down. He was born in August, and the days were hot. I vowed that day that I would never nurse him or any other baby of mine under a blanket. It's way too easy for them to have a heat stroke under a blanket on a sweltering day. I blame a society that insists that breastfeeding is shameful and that breastfeeding babies need to be hidden from the world.

> *Breastfeeding is a proud and loving act between mother and baby, and it is your baby's human right to nurse everywhere.*

WHY NOT COLD THERAPY?

Although Western medicine has promoted ice chips during labor, cold apple juice as a postpartum drink, and ice packs on the vulva after birth, this is taboo in African American postpartum culture because it is the opposite of what we know creates wellness during the postpartum period. We come from a hot continent, and our culture is one of warmth, hugs, and heat, which brings oxygen and nutrients to areas to promote healing, relax the muscles, and reduce inflammation. The mother must be protected from getting chills and being exposed to dampness, as the primary goal is to stay warm and dry for optimal healing.

Warming the mother should also include both her heart and body. An emotionally warm mother is more relaxed and more likely to maintain proper oxytocin levels because she feels loved and cared for. By keeping new mothers physically warm, you can help maintain their healthy immune system, prevent chills, and arm them against depression and mental confusion.

> *Your goal during the postpartum period is to stay warm and cozy. Keep a blanket on you, and keep your slippers nearby. Drink warm or at least room-temperature teas. Follow the example of our Granny Midwife ancestors, who knew how to help new mothers recover fully from childbirth.*

WARMTH WITH HYDROTHERAPY

Warm water is an important element in postpartum healing. After you've given birth, bonded with your baby, nursed them, had some nourishing postpartum soup, and feel strong enough to stand and walk, you can begin your water ritual. The most common is a hot shower, followed by a hot bath. Vaginal steaming, hot compresses, or warm sitz baths are all wonderful ways to bring heat to your body. These hydrotherapy practices should begin on day one, after you have eaten and slept; although some mamas opt to shower before they sleep. Using the traditions of our African ancestors, I give new mothers the traditional postpartum hot bath to heat the body up, relax the mother's muscles, and reduce pain in the vulva area.[8] Along with the warmth of the hot water, the steam from baths also helps increase breastmilk supply.[9]

If you've had a vaginal birth, you can take a hot Epsom salt bath at any time during your postpartum period to ease body aches. If you've had a cesarean birth, you should check with your medical provider before doing any water rituals. However, if you're cleared, you can wrap a hot water bottle in a towel or a heated rice sock and gently place it on or near your incision.

THE DELAYED BATHING TREND

A small movement is brewing, claiming that water cleansing, or bathing, right after birth is overrated and not needed. In the Western medical world, they tell new mothers to avoid washing their baby after birth, and some say that the postpartum bath for the mother should be delayed for three days or more. Daily bathing and a clean environment trace back to the great dynasties of Africa, like the Nubian and Khemet (Egyptian) empires, and in many Asian cultures as well. Remember, the number one practice that reduces disease is proper hygiene.

A Bathing Ritual

Another warming method is to create a hot steaming bathroom and instruct the new mother to sit in a tub of very warm medicinal water that covers her vulva, anal region, pelvis, and lower back, for immediate relief after birth. To create this steaming postpartum bath, start by washing the tub and filling it with extremely hot water. As you run the hot water, keep the bathroom door closed and cover any spaces around it to heat the bathroom. If the bathroom is still cold after running the hot water, you can use a space heater to help warm the room. In the meantime, boil a quart of water, then steep a cup of ginger root, a cup of comfrey root, and a cup of rosemary leaves. Be sure to pour a glass of room-temperature water for the mama as well. Though we want her to be warm, we do not want her to overheat or become dehydrated, so she needs to have something to drink while in the steamy bathroom and sitting in very warm water.

When the tub is one-third full, turn off the hot water and add the quart of strained herbal water. Once the tub is ready, set out some large cotton towels so the mother can dry off afterward. Depending on the size of the bathroom, you could light two to three unscented candles to help heat the bath and add soft light, which adds to the new mother's mental relaxation.

Once the postpartum bathwater is cool enough for the mother to sit in, make sure she puts on her robe, slippers, and hair bonnet and walk her to the bathroom. Close the door immediately after entering the bathroom to keep the heat in. Help her into the tub and place a warm, folded towel over her shoulders to prevent her from becoming chilled. The water should go up to her navel. Then, leave the mother alone for three to four minutes so she can relax, meditate, cry, or do whatever she feels like doing in privacy. Once she's had a few moments to herself, wash her back with warm water only, no soap. This will help her shoulders relax even more. Then, help her stand up and step out of the tub onto a dry nonslip rug, not a cold floor. Help her dry her body while keeping a towel over her shoulders to keep her warm. Then, help her put on her underwear and pad and support her as she gets redressed.

At this point, the new mother will be glistening with beauty from her postpartum medicinal bath. She has been steamed, soaked, washed, hydrated, and kept warm, and the smell of ginger, comfrey, and rosemary will help her body smell so fresh. This is a healing combination of both aromatherapy and hydrotherapy.

Afterward, be sure to help the mother back in the bed and cover her with warm blankets if the season requires it. She will likely fall into a deep sleep until the baby wakes her to nurse.

WARMING MASSAGES

Human touch is one of the most powerful conduits for creating and distributing heat to another human being. Direct touch or placing our hands three to five inches above the wounded areas, sore breasts and nipples, painful cesarean wounds, and/or sore joints can create the needed heat. Some refer to this method as Reiki. For postpartum mothers, massage is an important part of traditional care because it is the human exchange of energy that creates healing between two people: the giver and the receiver. The Granny Midwife followed the ancient custom of massaging new mothers, using goose grease, lard, coconut oil, and other types of available oils and greases. When I visited Senegal, I witnessed mothers massaging their pregnant daughters and grandbabies with lots of shea butter. Massaging also helps improve blood circulation, which increases the level of oxygen to the body. In our healing tradition, we help mama move toward whole-body wellness; therefore, while the massage helps heal sore parts, it is healing to the mind, body, and spirit as well. Rubbing mothers with warming oils is another way to honor them and show love and support.

There is no wrong time to give a postpartum massage, but I like to offer a fifteen- to twenty-minute massage after a postpartum medicinal bath because the mother is already relaxed and her muscles have been softened by the warm bathwater.

How to Massage a New Mama

- Massage mama in her bed so she doesn't have to move around before or after.
- Choose and prepare your oil. Massage oil should always be safe for the baby. I use edible oils, such as olive oil, coconut oil, shea butter, tallow, sesame oil, and general vegetable oil.
- Place a half cup of oil in a small stainless-steel pot and warm the oil over exceptionally low heat. The goal is for the oil to be warmed, not hot.
- After the oil is warm, turn off the stove and put a lid on the pot to keep the heat in. Transfer the oil into a ceramic or glass bowl. I always check the heat of the oil on my inner arm.
- Two cautions:

  * Do not warm the oil in the microwave, as it can become too hot and can burn the mother, infant, or you.
  * For the sake of the baby, I do not recommend adding

essential oils to your homemade postpartum massage oil or using premade postpartum oils that have been infused with essential oils.

- When your oil is prepared, wash your hands with hot, soapy water. The hotter the water, the warmer your hands will be for the massage.
- Set your intention. I set my intention by saying an internal prayer, similar to the Granny Midwives, asking the Creator to help my work please God and be acceptable to our fellow man, and I add, "Let my hands be a blessing and a comfort to the mother."[10]
- Next, rub your hands together to create energy; this further warms them up. You should not touch a postpartum mother with cold hands.
- Moderately coat your right palm with the oil, then rub your palms together to distribute the oil equally and warm your hands up. You can also pour about two teaspoons of warmed oil onto the mother's back and distribute it equally. The lower back is a great place to start.
- Once you've applied the oil, gently rub on mama's back, move up to her upper back and massage her shoulders because that is where worry often sits.
- Other areas to massage for warming are the abdomen, breasts, and the feet. After you gently massage the breasts, you can apply very warm facecloths to help keep milk flowing.
- Before you wrap up, ask mama if there are any particular areas that she wants massaged.
- When finished, wrap mama up in blankets so she stays warm, and let her lie in bed to rest.

Additional Tip: Regularly check in with mama during the massage to ensure she does not feel pain and wants you to continue massaging.

SACRED WARMTH

The postpartum period is a sacred time for mama and baby to cuddle with good, warm foods and cozy blankets. We want mama to feel completely protected and comfortable, which releases the necessary hormones for postpartum health and full recuperation.

Warming Tips

- Cultivate warming as a practice—warm the environment, your body, and your newborn's body.
- Utilize wet and dry heat, and be creative with your methods—baths, warm wet compresses, touch, blankets, space heaters, warm foods and teas, hot water bottles, warmed rice socks, etc.
- Practice the rituals of skin-to-skin contact, postpartum baths, and massages as soon after birth as possible.
- Blankets make great mother shower blessing gifts. New moms need at least five blankets to cycle through when one becomes soiled. Natural fabrics warm best. Because they can be spendy, they make a great joint gift for a family.
- Wear slippers.
- In the hospital, request warm blankets. They will be just the right temperature to help you relax. You can request as many warming blankets as you need during your postpartum hospital stay.

- Once you're home, continue to use warm blankets. You can warm blankets by placing them in the dryer on low heat for twenty-five to thirty minutes. Make sure the blanket is free of metals, like zippers and clips, because the metal will heat up and can burn you or your infant.

You can help yourself have a positive postpartum experience by staying warm. Let your postpartum environment be like a warm hug from a loved one.

CHAPTER 5

Cleansed

We give thanks to the Creator for the power and blessings of the water that sustains life and helps our babies grow in the womb. Thank you for the heavenly rain as the purifier and nourisher of Mother Earth, and of body and mind.

Bless this new mother with soothing, nourishing water. May she be purified and sanctified during her transition into motherhood. May her newborn be blessed and cleansed. Let water be healing to her body and soul, let it keep her free from infection, and allow her to feel cleansed, anointed, and beautiful. Amen.

I LOVED GROWING UP IN ALABAMA WITH MY GRANDMOTHER, A foot-washing Baptist who cleansed her feet in a basin of warm water every night before saying her prayers and getting into bed. To many African Americans, water is considered sacred, and cleanliness is holy. When my grandmother saw the sky filling with rain clouds, she would give us directions to bring out the wash tubs. These were six-gallon metal tubs that people would bathe or wash their clothes in. We would place the two tubs in the middle of the yard, and the rainwater that would fill them up was considered holy and purified because it came down from the heavens.

A small portion of the rainwater would be stored in bottles for hair rinsing because rainwater is believed to make your hair grow healthier. Freshly washed bed sheets would be put in the tub of rain water, swished around a few times, rung out, and then hung on the clotheslines to dry. The hot Alabama sun dried the sheets in less than thirty minutes, bleaching them a brilliant white. To this day, I remember how fresh they smelled of sun and rain as I pulled them off the clothesline and put them in the basket to make up the beds. Lying on the fragrant sheets always put me in a deep and restful sleep.

My grandmother was born in late 1895. She still had direct knowledge of African ways and had assisted Granny Midwives with births and postpartum care. She passed down to me the African concept of staying clean all throughout life, including during pregnancy, afterbirth, and postpartum. She showed me that cleaning and being cleansed was a tradition, a responsibility, a religion, and a culture. My grandma was meticulous. She taught many cleansing rituals around our food, home, environment, and bodies. She drilled in us grandchildren the value of hygiene and maintaining clean surroundings, thoughts, and speech.

A common African American saying is that "Cleanliness is next to godliness." The most important vehicle for cleansing in our culture is water because it is rooted in our ancestral understanding of water as a source of life and a vehicle for purification, rejuvenation, beautification, healing, and regeneration. In Black culture, water is said to purify the body, spirit, mind, and environment. I was taught that cleaning and being cleansed were spiritual acts and a way to anoint yourself and others.

The sacredness of water doesn't just stop here, though. It is demonstrated in various religions where water is used in ceremony. In Christian baptisms, believers are dunked in or anointed by water to be cleansed of their sins and reborn. In Islam, practitioners must wash particular areas of the body before they can pray, and women must bathe after their menses ends and after sexual intercourse. In Catholicism, priests bless the water before it is used to make the sign of the cross. In Hinduism, the Ganges River is considered sacred and is believed to heal ailments. And the Yoruba religion, one of the many spiritual paths of West Africa, deeply respects the water as sacred, personifying it with the revered Orisha Yemaya, who represents the sea, motherhood, and nurturing energy.

As such, cleansing is one of the core principles of postpartum care. This is a time when new mothers are experiencing physiological changes that carry the risk of infection and involve bodily fluids, like sweat, blood, urine, and leaking milk. She deserves to feel fresh, revived, and attractive during this beautiful and challenging time. The core principles of purification also help restore harmony to her emotions, which can be greatly affected during the postpartum period.

Many African American postpartum cleansing practices include water, dry rubs, oils, clays, and steams to cleanse the five senses. These include methods of washing the birthing areas to help it heal, allowing the mother to soak in shallow herbal baths or sitz baths for relaxation, pouring bowls of warm water over the vaginal area after using the bathroom for quick relief, or vaginal steaming to promote healing. It's also customary to use gentle soaps on the upper parts of the mother's body or use citrus fruits, like lemons, limes, and orange peels to scrub the entire body. Submerging in a bath, standing under a shower, or taking a sponge bath are all parts of this ritual of cleansing as well.

As we honor the mother in holistic ways with thorough and consistent cleansing, we bring in ancient traditions and science to keep her free from infection and disease and improve her mood.

Cleansing rituals and practices serve as a celebratory recognition for the achievement of birth. Being cleansed with water helps protect the body, mind, and environment from negative energy and regenerates energy. As a new mother, you deserve a clean body and environment. And when you have a stressful, long, or physically active day, you can use water to cleanse yourself and restore equilibrium. Being cleansed will help you re-center your emotions and feel your best.

The Cleansing Power of Fire

Fire and heat are other aspects of African American cleansing and postpartum traditions. In addition to using water, we also heat, burn, and smoke things to cleanse them. When it was time to take the mother out of bed after her forty-two days of focused care, the first thing the Granny Midwife would do was smoke the mother's first outdoor outfit. These practices can be traced to several African postpartum rituals, where the mother's clothes were smoked with a special scented wood to purify them. When the new mother reentered the community, her special smell preceded her, and the community knew by the fragrance that she was coming out.

In the twentieth-century South, the Granny Midwives used corn for this smoking ritual, but today, there are other options. You can even get resin imported from parts of Africa.

To smoke a mother's clothes, I put frankincense and myrrh resin crystals on red-hot charcoal in a firesafe burner in the bathroom. I dampen the mother's clothes by wetting my hands and wiping them on her dress. Then, using a hanger, I hang the dress on the shower rod or towel rack. I then get the bathroom nice and smoky with the resin smoke and shut the door, leaving *the clothes to smoke overnight. This allows the clothes to hold a stronger, longer-lasting smell. If a new mother feels strong at forty-two days postpartum and she has no help, she can smoke her own clothes. This ritual represents the sweet and high status of motherhood.*

Sometimes, we also smoke the birthing room to purify it with regional herbs or according to the family's practice. I do not use sage to cleanse my postpartum homes because sage has been overharvested in the twenty-first century. I decline its use out of respect for the environment[1] and also because it can dry breast-milk.[2] Instead, I use what I call the "Baby Jesus gifts": frankincense and myrrh. Both are antibacterial, helping to cleanse both the air and objects.

CLEANSING TO SUPPORT POSTPARTUM PHYSIOLOGICAL CHANGES

I remember visiting three Granny Midwives while attending a Black midwives retreat in Houston, Texas. I had my third baby with me, who was almost four months old at the time. He began crying, and I pulled out my breast to nurse him as I had with all my children. The Granny Midwives looked at me surprised, and one said, "Ain't you going to wash off your breast?" Of course, I said, "Yes, ma'am," because I duly respected them and always did what they said. I did not ask why I should, nor did they say explain why or where this tradition came from. I went into the bathroom and used water to wash my breast on the sides, all the way to my armpit. Then I returned to sit with them and nursed my baby like normal.

In all of my travel and conference attending, I had never heard that a mother should wash her breast before nursing. I was taught that a mother's breast was automatically clean and did not need any preparation, and in fact putting soap on the nipple would dry it out, so I never did it. However, a year later, I attended a birth where the newborn would not nurse. Everything appeared fine with the baby, and it was clear she wanted to nurse because she was rooting and smacking her lips, but something was stopping her and she began to get fussy. We tried several methods, but her baby would not latch on to her breast. I considered myself an expert in this work, but nothing I tried worked. I even attempted to nurse the baby myself—with mama's permission, of course—to see if she knew how to suck, and she successfully latched on to my breast.

Then, I remembered what I learned from the Granny Midwives in Texas. I asked the mother to let me wash her breasts with water and a dab of soap under her armpits. When she offered her breast to her infant, the baby latched on like there had never been a problem. We realized that the baby did not like the smell of her mother's armpits from perspiring during labor. I witnessed firsthand the benefits of being cleansed and specifically washing the breast and underarms before nursing. Listening to my elders taught me something that, to this day, I have never read in a breastfeeding book or heard in a breastfeeding lecture.

From leaking breastmilk to baby and mama's various bodily fluids, there are so many reasons a postpartum home calls for cleansing. Let's look at some of the physiological reasons:

Sweat

A pregnant woman, on average, gains about twenty-five to thirty-five pounds, depending on her age, body type, the number of babies in her womb, and other indicators. At least three pounds of this weight is extra fluid in the body, which often shows up as swelling during pregnancy, especially in the second and third trimesters. This extra fluid leaves the body during the postpartum period through increased urination and perspiration. Often referred to as night sweats or hot flashes, this is reported by 29 percent of new mothers.[3] Night sweats are most noticeable in the first two weeks but can happen for the first six weeks postpartum.

Hormones like estrogen, progesterone, and relaxin remain elevated during pregnancy and drop significantly after birth while oxytocin and prolactin increase. This change in hormones can also cause increased sweating postpartum, usually at night.[4] I remember waking up with my first baby at twenty-one years old, all wet from sweating, and thinking to myself, *What is happening?* Then, I was informed that my body was ridding itself of excess water and regulating its hormones, and it all started to make sense. After that night, I made a habit of getting in the shower regularly, and when I did, I always felt so much better. Of course, I also went through quite a few new gowns and bed sheets!

What You Can Do If You Have Night Sweats

- Use cotton sheets with a 180–280 thread count, as these are the most breathable.
- Change the sheets as often as needed.
- Drink plenty of water to stay hydrated.
- Take daily showers, baths, or sponge baths to refresh yourself.
- Wipe your body with peppermint water.
- Wear natural, breathable fabrics, such as light cotton gowns.
- Bathe your baby regularly, especially if you co-sleep.

Postpartum Bleeding, or Lochia

After the delivery of your placenta, you will start the postpartum bleeding process with red bleeding called rubra. By day ten, it will change to a pinkish discharge called alba. And for the remaining twenty days, it will become a yellowish-white discharge called serosa. During this time, use only dye- and perfume-free organic pads—no tampons or menstrual cups until after those first six weeks. The cervix takes ten days to close, so absolutely nothing should enter your vagina until it closes.

How to Cleanse Yourself:

- Take daily showers, baths, or sponge baths.
- Change your pad every two hours or when it feels uncomfortable.
- A good timekeeper is to change your sanitary pad every time you use the bathroom, depending on how bloody it is.
- Urine, lochia, and blood are a medium for bacteria, so you should always wipe front to back, drop the toilet paper, then wipe again from front to back until you are clean.
- Use the peri squeeze bottle from the hospital to rinse your vaginal area with warm water. This helps keep the area clean and makes you feel better.
- Add rose water or orange blossom to your peri bottle to feel fresh and provide a natural fragrance.
- Change soiled panties regularly.
- Wash your hands with soap and water whenever you change your pad.

Note: If you are soaking a pad in an hour or are passing blood clots the size of a large egg, contact your doctor ASAP or go directly to the emergency room. If you feel dizzy or weak while bleeding, call 911 right away. While waiting for the ambulance, lie flat, elevate your feet above your heart, and put a blanket over you. This can prevent you from going into shock from blood loss.

Warming and Cleansing

The postpartum herbal warming bath I shared in chapter 4 is also an opportunity to cleanse yourself. As the water warms you, you are also being cleansed by the herbs in the bath. The traditional African American cleansing methods include water, steam, sand, dry sauna, oils, and hot water, so feel free to use whatever methods feel right to you. I always encourage new mothers to cleanse themselves with water and a little natural soap each morning to cleanse the skin of any nighttime perspiration or breastmilk. Over the years, I have heard many mothers comment about how clammy their skin felt, which made them feel uncomfortable. This is the result of lingering sweat on the skin. If you're concerned about dry skin from bathing often, you can always oil your breasts and body with a non-fragrant vegetable oil as needed.

CLEANSING THE POSTPARTUM SPACE

African American postpartum cleansing is not just about a clean body; it's also about a clean environment. A clean postpartum environment prevents the spread of infection, reduces chaos, and promotes peace for the entire household. Keeping the home clean physically and spiritually helps mothers manage their postpartum emotions better and keeps family members in good spirits. Granny Midwives told us to wash up daily. This tradition and discipline remains one of the foundations to reducing stress in motherhood and later in life. Healthy habits help sustain a positive environment in the home, so the mother can end her six weeks and begin moving about with ease. The tradition of being and staying clean is a life skill. I taught my seven children—three sons and four daughters—these skills, and they all said it benefited them while living in a college dorm, being a roommate, living alone, and on the job.

When cleaning your environment, consider using organic, nontoxic cleaning supplies. Most home surfaces can be cleaned with a mild soap and warm water. There are many things on the market that are considered safe as well as some basic things you may already have in your kitchen, like water, lemons, white vinegar, baking soda, and a neutral oil to polish furniture. My grandmother always said, "You welcome your guests into a clean home." A clean house is a great way to welcome the new mother and her baby.

Plants as Cleansing

Indoor plants are important to have around, as they bring in good energy and improve indoor air quality.

- Potted indoor plants reduce CO_2 in the home, improve air quality,[5] boost people's well-being,[6] decrease indoor noise, and limit the amount of dust particles in the air.
- Having fresh flowers throughout the house adds visual beauty, reduces tension, and increases relaxation.[7] Be

sure to remove dead flowers from bouquets, snip the stems weekly, change the water daily, and add sugar to the water to keep the flowers healthy. Wilting or dead-looking bouquets can drain positive energy, so if the bouquet is dead, toss it and bring in a new one.

The Queen's Room

It's important that the mother's postpartum room stays clean and fresh. When cleaning, be sure to take the baby out of the room, as some cleansing products are too pungent for their sensitive system. Here are a few things you can do to keep mama's room feeling light and smelling good:

- Air out the room daily by opening windows, weather permitting.
- Wash floors with vinegar, lemon, or essential oils.
- Use herbs like frankincense, myrrh, or sandalwood to purify the air.
- Use an air purifier.
- Keep at least three to five potted plants in the room.
- Wipe frequently handled items with alcohol wipes, lemon, vinegar, diluted tea tree or rosemary oil, soap, and water. All of these work to remove dirt and germs, and are natural antiseptics and antifungal agents.
- Change the bed sheets and pillowcases, and be sure to use natural fibers (cotton or linen). Research confirms that natural, breathable fabrics are best for our skin.[8] This is especially important to keep in mind if you co-sleep with your baby, as their skin is incredibly sensitive.

The Importance of Hygiene with Clothing and Shoes

- Never sit on mama's bed while wearing outside clothes because this is where the mother resides with the newborn. The elders believed that you could transfer outside germs on the bed, and they were certainly right!
- Use a changing pad or baby blanket beneath the baby whenever you change their diaper. This prevents any bacteria from getting directly on surfaces. Babies always seem to urinate once their diaper is off.
- Never put outside shoes on any furniture, especially the bed or sofa. The soles of our shoes are filthy. We walk through garbage, animal and human waste, phlegm, and who knows what else when we step outside. This is why, in some cultures, shoes are left outside the door before entering the house.
- Keep an extra set or two of clean bed sheets available at all times so you can change them as soon as they are soiled.

CLEANING TIPS

My mother always said, "Messy isn't dirty." That meant having clean clothes on the sofa for folding, rinsed dishes stacked for the dishwasher, or toys and books lying around is acceptable. What is unacceptable is unemptied garbage cans, dirty plates, pots of old food, unswept floors, bathtub and sink rings, and dirty toilets.

Simple Cleaning Supplies to Have on Hand

- Broom, dust pan, mop, vacuum cleaner with HEPA filter bags, buckets, garbage bags, disposable gloves, cleaning liquids, and a washer and dryer

- Sponges, cotton cloths, paper towels, toilet paper, tub cleaner, dish-washing liquid, and liquids for the dish-washer, if there is one
- Air filter for pollen and pollution
- Unscented detergent and natural dryer sheets, if you use them
- A minimum of one set of bed sheets, which includes a fit-ted sheet, a top sheet, and one clean pillowcase for every pillow on the bed
- Three large cotton terry towels and hand soap (not hand sanitizer)
- Some families invest in paper plates to avoid having to wash dishes. This is certainly great for convenience; however, the mother is the queen, so I serve her food on porcelain or ceramic plates.

When I make postpartum home visits, I like to bring my apron because it allows me to keep all the items I'll need on hand to serve the mother better, such as disposable gloves, body salves, tea bags, and my phone. I always enter mama's home with good intentions to be of service, bring peace and joy, and support her in bonding with her baby.

When I enter the house, I remove my outside shoes and put on my inside shoes. I say a prayer and ask that my intuition be strong enough to fill in for any unspoken needs, and I ask that the mother, baby, and family be blessed with good health and harmony. Once the mother is nourished with food and hydration, I help her bathe, shower, or wash up at the sink, depending on her choice. She should eat and drink before being cleansed to make sure she has the strength to participate in the rituals. After the mother is bathed and dressed in clean clothes, I prop her feet up and give her something to drink, usually raspberry leaf, ginger root, nettle, blueberry leaf, and mint leaf tea with honey. While she sips her tea and relaxes from her bath, I change and wash her bed linen, and if the baby has a bed or changing table, I change and wash those too. If there are enough baby clothes, I wash them separately. I love cleaning the mother's room to raise the energetic vibrations and see her smile. She always appreciates the attention and care.

When I'm done, I ask mama if she wants to return to bed. If so, I put down a pad to protect her sheets, usually in the first and second week postpartum, then I take about a fifteen- to twenty-minute break. With the mother's permission, I like to put on quiet instrumental music while I clean the rest of the home. After I finish with the mother's room, emptying any trash, removing leftover food, sweeping or vacuuming if needed, freshening flowers, watering plants, cracking windows or doors for fresh air, or ensuring the room stays warm, I then put a pitcher of water and a cup on mama's nightstand so she can access water as needed. I also give her a small bowl of either fruit, cubes of cut chicken, room-temperature black-eyed peas, or a boiled egg cut in half to snack on. After mama is back in bed, I hold the baby or wrap them on my back African-style if they need attention so mama can get more sleep.

My job is to make sure the mother and baby are physically clean and feel their best. I leave the cleaning of the general home area, such as the front room, dining room, and other children's bedrooms for the rest of the mother's helpers.

GETTING CLEANING SUPPORT

For help with household chores, I encourage you to call on old and new friends, check with your faith communities to see if they have a Visiting the Sick program, or ask your sorority sisters if they can provide maternity care support. Ask extended family and adolescent children for help. Keep a list of needs taped to the refrigerator, or make a Google Doc and send it to family and friends. Offer simple directions and many thank-yous.

If you don't have adequate support, do not try to do everything on your own. Ignore the messiness of your house and tell yourself that it is only temporary and your rest is more important. Remember, you need all the energy you can get to take care of yourself and your baby. Take it slow during your lying-in period. The first six weeks of postpartum will be over before you know it, and by then, you'll have the energy and strength to take on some of the chores.

Cleansing Your Newborn

I remember visiting a postpartum mother whose baby constantly cried with seemingly no relief in sight. I ran the tub full of warm water and submerged the baby up to his neck, so his entire body was in the water. I supported the baby's head with my hands as he floated in the water. I left the lights off and ensured the room was warm. After five minutes of letting the baby float, I took him out and wrapped him in a large white terry towel rather than a blanket. Miraculously, the baby was completely calm and cleansed of his stress. Mama was then able to nurse him to sleep. By cleaning the newborn with warm water, I was able to help him relax and stop crying.

New mama, you have birthed and been birthed as a new mother. Take your postpartum period as a renewal, as a spiritual and physical cleansing. Embark on your new path with joy and commit yourself to rituals of care, hygiene, beautification, and a cleansed environment. You deserve it.

CHAPTER 6

Nourished

God, thank you for this food. We ask you to bless this food, those who grew it, and those who prepared it. May the power of this food, energized by the sun, bring nourishment to the mother, who labored hard to birth her baby. May this food create smiles, laughter, healing, and love.

May you be satiated, energized, and warmed by the food you eat. May you be served and honored through food. May it bring you peace, higher vibrations, and good healing. Let the colors, aromas, tastes, and textures delight and support you. Let your food represent community and togetherness during your post-partum period. May you feel connected to the history of your ancestors and the foods we grew, prepared, and ate. Amen.

BY THE TIME MY SECOND BABY WAS BORN, I WAS BETTER VERSED in Black postpartum traditions. In September, there were still plenty of fresh vegetables and fruits being harvested, and I remember lying in bed with my baby, listening to my sisters and husband laughing as they cooked for me in the kitchen. Each week, they made me something new to eat over the next two to three days.

For the first week, they made me a light soup with a tomato base, red palm oil, fish, shrimp, black-eyed peas, okra, onion, sea salt, and dashes of cayenne. Rice or cornmeal was the main starch that always accompanied the meals. Even though the soup was "light," it was delicious and very fulfilling. Then, they made turnip greens and palm oil stews, with all parts of a chicken included, and simmered peanut soup with goat meat and bones until the goat was tender. Later, they added in sweet potatoes and seasoned it all with onion, salt, smoked paprika, cumin, and black pepper. For a snack, they gently fried chicken livers in butter and served them on crackers, and I ate that twice weekly. In between, I was fed savory soft cornbread with black strap molasses poured over it and a glass of room-temperature buttermilk. Week three was the same tomato-base soup with goat, green peas, and chopped turnip greens. Week four was gumbo with seafood, smoked turkey necks, celery, thyme, white potatoes, bay leaf, bell peppers, tomatoes, and black-eyed peas.

This pattern continued for the first forty-two days. Once we all finished the soup, family and visitors included, my sister would repeat the soup base and add different ingredients, like chicken, collard greens, turnips, or sweet potatoes. In the morning, I was usually fed a small bowl of loose grits with cheese, salt, black pepper, butter, and soft scrambled eggs. There was a lot of cornbread, bananas, sliced apples, cups of buttermilk, and hot herbal postpartum teas, mostly ginger, raspberry, and dandelion with a little honey during the day and chamomile and catnip in the evening to help me sleep. After the six weeks were completed, I continued eating a diet high in organ meats and leafy, green vegetables.

Like my grandma and the women of her era, my sisters could throw down delicious, nutritious Southern meals. They used fresh vegetables, cooked from scratch, and could have it all done, including dessert, in thirty minutes if company showed up unexpectedly. My grandma used to keep a jar of hot peppers marinated in vinegar with black peppercorn and cloves ready at all times. And like our African ancestors, she had a go-to one-pot meal that was usually stewed in its own juices. By sautéing the seasoning, folding in salted and peppered flour, and stirring until brown, using the juice from the meats and vegetables, she could come up with brown gravy for rice or cornbread that contained the protein and nutrients of everything that had been cooked.

Food has long been considered medicine in our community, with common sayings, like "You are what you eat," "Health is wealth," and "Do not waste food." For generations now, prominent Black folks have written about the power of food as medicine. In the early 1900s, George Washington Carver researched the health benefits of peanuts; in the 1930s, the Honorable Elijah Muhammad wrote *How to Eat to Live*, which includes concepts and recipes for using food as a source of mental power, improved physical appearance and health, and longevity; in 1971, in her book *The African Heritage Cookbook*, Helen Mendes discussed the deep connection to the land that began with our African ancestors and was carried forward by Black Southern farmers; and many modern chefs, scholars, and writers continue to reclaim our food ways and traditions, including Adrian Miller, Toni Tipton-Martin, Michael W. Twitty, Dr. Deborah Harris, Bryant Terry, Stephen Satterfield, and the art collective Ghetto Gastro. We have a vibrant food culture that has been passed down through oral and firsthand traditions, celebrating our historical links with Africa and honoring the ways we use food—growing, cooking, baking, and consuming it—for medicinal, spiritual, social, and political purposes.

Whether they are from the Caribbean, Africa, or North or South America, Black people around the globe have visceral experiences with food; there is a cellular recognition that food heals. Having the ability to access, prepare, and eat your cultural foods is all part of its healing power. The idea that food is medicine can be traced back to early African civilizations, where people valued the produce that came from the land, not only for enjoyment and community-building, but also for maintaining good health. This knowledge was passed down to African Americans by their enslaved African ancestors, who taught them to be stewards of the land, grow organic food for the sake of their health, and pay homage to the Creator for the sustenance. Today, science has confirmed what these ancestors knew centuries ago: Food is our first and best medicine, starting with the milk from our mothers.

Through research and oral stories from older women both in the American South and Africa, I learned that new mothers were given iron-rich foods after birth, such as dandelion leaves and collards, stewed organ meats, and bones, to help boost their health and vitality. Mamas were often given stir-fried chicken livers served with brown gravy and rice, lots of dark green vegetables, and plenty of soups and stews made with tomatoes, bell pepper, peas, okra, poultry, fish, and meat. These recipes were said to restore their strength, protect them from illness, and give them an abundant supply of healthy breastmilk. Once I learned this, I made sure to feed every mother I assisted as a midwife at least one African American postpartum meal. It is tradition, and I am a traditionalist. When I hear news of a new baby, I remind the family to cook our cultural postpartum recipes for the mother and bake at least one cake or pie to celebrate the occasion.

We call our food "spiritual food," and that has many meanings, but the most profound meaning is that food heals the mind, body, and soul. The rich and nutritious African American postpartum diet gets its foundation from the nutrient-dense foods of the African continent. Before colonization, Africa was comprised of advanced empires, kingdoms, chiefdoms, nations, regions, and large families/clans, and all of these groups were descendants of hunters and gatherers, nomads, herders, fishers, and farmers. When the people from these distinct communities were kidnapped and put onto plantations together, their dietary patterns evolved into the unique African American diet, which maintained the African foundations of one-pot meals, soups, and stews. These dietary influences can be traced to Ghana, Nigeria, Burundi, Zanzibar, Congo, Kenya, Ethiopia, Dahomey, Chad, and Guinea.[1] And our foundational foods include beans, peas, rice, sweet potatoes, okra, corn, hot peppers, leafy greens, root vegetables, fermented foods, and a variety of fruits, like watermelon, coconut, peaches, bananas, and grapes.

The Granny Midwives knew that healthy, organic food promoted optimal physical and mental health, and that it had to be respected for its medicinal powers to be released. Each food group offers special healing for the body because they each contain a different composition of protein, vitamins, and minerals. Combining them with intention and in the right balance makes their medicine stronger. According to the Granny Midwife, certain plants come to those who need them as a food source, even when a person is unaware that they need a particular nutrient. For instance, chickweed contains protein, amino acids, vitamins, and minerals. When the midwife noticed that chickweed had taken over her front yard, she assumed that she needed those nutrients and began adding it to her diet. Similarly, when a postpartum mother requests a particular food from a specific category, it is believed that she needs the nutrients or medicine from that particular food.

Nourishment through quality foods is fundamental for a full recuperation from pregnancy, birth, and breastfeeding. The food you consume during your postpartum period plays a vital role in determining your future health and well-being and your ability to care for your baby and yourself. Food can either be a medicine or a poison, so it is important to consume foods that heal the body.

The purpose of food in the Black postpartum tradition is to nourish the body and uplift the emotions. Intent matters, ingredients matter, and who cooks it and how matters. Whole-body nourishment is a core part of Black postpartum care, and feeding a new mother well is a noble act. When we nourish the mother, we honor the female body and reclaim our African foodways. Reacquainting ourselves with these foods and learning how to cook them from scratch is a powerful reclamation of our ancestral methods for thriving.

SPIRITUAL FOOD FOR POSTPARTUM CARE

The first thing many new mothers say after greeting their new baby is, "I am starving." The body uses many calories during labor and childbirth—at least three hundred calories per hour. Although the postpartum period is not a time of illness, it is a crucial time for you to consume nutritious food to recover from the loss of nutrients during pregnancy and labor. Hunger inhibits your ability to think, sleep, tolerate pain, and ease anxiety and depression. The purpose of nourishment in the postpartum period is to give your body the vitamins, minerals, proteins, and probiotics it needs to recover from ten lunar months of pregnancy, labor, and birth, and heal the placenta site. It is also an essential component to produce quality and abundant breastmilk. It's essential that food is kept front and center during the entire postpartum period so you can meet both your body's visible and invisible needs.

Your visible signs of health include regaining strength or even an acknowledgment that you feel better. The invisible signs will be shown through bloodwork and your vital signs, including blood pressure, blood sugar, and urine (this can show if bacteria are present or if your white blood cell count is high, which are signs of infection). Food's "invisible work" is in providing you with enough calories to maintain your energy and strength, regenerating new cells to repair internal injuries (vaginal tears, placenta wound, fat stores replacement), and rebuilding your iron supplies and immune system to fight off infections.

Postpartum nourishment should be delicious, wet, warm, spicy, fatty, and nutrient dense. Dietary fat is important because research shows it helps with hormone regulation, maternal brain restoration, and energy production, which helps mama heal well and care for her newborn.[2] Healthy saturated fats can be obtained from any meat product as well as coconut oil, butter, palm oil, and raw peanut oil. The Granny Midwives also used lard, tallow, or goose grease mixed with herbs to heal cracked nipples, vaginal tears, hemorrhoids, diaper rash, and cradle cap and perform postpartum massages. Fat should be consumed daily during the lying-in period or until lactation ends.

African American postpartum meals typically include porridges, soups, stews, gravies, rice dishes, meat and poultry, organ meats, puddings, and hot herbal drinks. The Granny Midwife's taboo postpartum foods include pork, cabbage, cold cuts, pasta, and any cold foods like ice cream, pasta salads, potato salads, and the like. She believed cabbage would give the mother and baby excess gas and stomach cramps, cold cuts were nutritionally empty, and pork was too high in sodium, causing headaches and high blood pressure.

Here are other key concepts to keep in mind for proper postpartum nourishment:

Use Blemish-Free, Organic Foods and Meats

If organic produce isn't in your budget, the next best choice is frozen foods, then sodium-free, organic, canned foods. Our ancestors mainly ate free-range meats and poultry and wild-caught fish, but do the best you can. Conventionally farmed animals are often pumped full of hormones and antibiotics, so try to avoid them when possible. Food deserts in Black communities are a real barrier to optimal food choices, but if you're able, find local (preferably Black-owned-and-operated) farmers' markets or practice urban gardening. You can also try telling your local grocery store that you need fresh, organic vegetables, or you can carpool with friends or family to shop outside your neighborhood.

The First Postpartum Meal Will Set the Tone

Just as a marathon runner grabs nourishment to start their recovery as soon as the race is over, a new mother must immediately begin replenishing her body after birth. I encourage the mother or her family to have at least one postpartum soup ready before birth so once the baby is born, the mother can be fed a nourishing warm soup and get her body moving toward regeneration right away.

If I'm assisting with a hospital birth, I pack a thermos of my chicken curry coconut soup and feed it to the mother once the medical provider says it is okay for her to have food and liquids. This meal helps soothe and nourish her mind and body because it has bone broth, fat, protein, a multitude of vitamins, and vinegar to help with calcium absorption. When I say "feed," I mean I hand-feed her soup with a spoon or put it in a coffee cup and hold it to her mouth so she can sip it. I also always stand in front of the mother so she doesn't have to turn her head to be fed; turning the neck causes neck pain and is bad for digestion. Before feeding her, I make sure mama is sitting up with her back fully supported to aid in proper digestion. If she's at home, I put enough pillows behind her so she can sit up comfortably.

Prioritize Iron-Rich Foods

When I was a teenager, I learned I had iron-deficient anemia. My doctor prescribed iron tablets, but he did not explain the seriousness of this disease to my daily well-being. When I became a midwife, I learned that iron-deficient anemia is a health condition characterized by insufficient red blood cells or hemoglobin. Hemoglobin is a protein that the body makes using iron to carry oxygen from the lungs to other body parts. As such, iron is an important part of the diet, as it is what keeps oxygen abundant in our bloodstream. Maintaining proper iron levels can be a challenge during pregnancy for several reasons, including poor diet, fetal development, preexisting iron deficiency, or blood disorders like sickle cell anemia or thalassemia. You may also need iron postpartum if you lose too much blood or have a massive hemorrhage during birth.

All postpartum mothers need to eat an iron-rich diet for the first twelve months postpartum. This is particularly important for mothers who had cesarean births or those who lost excessive amounts of blood during birth or early in the postpartum period. Mothers with low iron may experience a host of health problems that can be remedied by increasing their consumption of iron-rich foods and taking iron supplements.

The African American postpartum diet historically fed new mother innards or organ meats, like heart, liver, kidneys, and gizzards. While some people may find organ meats distasteful, eating them can help restore iron to your blood cells. You should eat organ meat twice weekly for at least the first twenty-four weeks postpartum.

If you're not interested in organ meats, be sure to consume a diverse diet so you know you're getting enough iron. Shellfish offers the highest amount of iron, followed by chicken livers, and goat meat. Chicken liver, in particular, is an easy source of absorbable iron. Vegetables and other plant-based foods contain nonheme (plant) iron, which has optimal absorption when accompanied by a source of vitamin C. Think of food combinations like oats and berries; grits and green peppers; lentils and sweet potatoes; spinach, tomatoes, and potatoes; kale and tomato sauce; or citrus juice squeezed on veggies and beans.

If you're pregnant, you need approximately twenty-seven milligrams of iron per day. If you're breastfeeding, your iron needs drop to nine milligrams per day. And if you are not breastfeeding, your nonpregnant iron needs are eighteen milligrams per day.[3]

HEME (ANIMAL MEAT) IRON	
Food	Iron per serving
Clams	24 mg per 3-oz serving
Oysters	7 to 9 mg per 3-oz serving
Sardines	4.4 mg per cup
Mussels	3 to 5 mg per 3.5-oz serving
Chicken liver	9 mg per 3-oz serving
Goat	3.2 mg per 3-oz serving
Chicken	1.5 mg per 3-oz serving
Shrimp	2.6 mg per 3-oz serving
Beef	2.9 mg per 3-oz serving

NONHEME (PLANT) IRON	
Blackstrap molasses	15 to 18 mg per 8-oz serving
Blackstrap molasses is not only rich in iron, but it also provides calcium, magnesium, and potassium, making it a great natural option for boosting nutrient intake.	
Fresh spearmint leaves	12 mg per 100 g
Cooked pumpkin leaves	3.2 mg per 100 g
Basil	2 mg per 3.5-oz serving
Beet greens	2.6 mg per 100 g
Cooked broccoli leaves	1.1 mg per 100 g (or 3.5-oz serving)
Dulse	8 mg per 100 g
Kelp (dried)	2.8 mg per 100 g
Cooked collard greens	2.5 mg per cup
Cooked dandelion greens	1.7 m per cup
Cooked kale	1.1 mg per cup (about 130 grams)
Cooked mustard greens	1.64 mg per 100 g (simmered and drained)
Romaine lettuce	0.97 mg per 100 g
Spinach	3.6 mg per 100 g
Lima beans	3.1 mg per 100 g
Black-eyed peas	2.2 mg per 100 g
Swiss chard	2.26 mg per 100 g
Turnips	1.15 mg per 100 g
Watercress	0.2 mg per 100 g
Navy beans	4.4 mg per 100 g
Peanuts (goobers)	4.6 mg per cup of raw peanuts (about 146 g)
Dried prunes	5 mg per cup (This is roughly 58 percent of the daily recommended intake.)
Okra	0.62 mg per cup (raw)
	0.4 mg per 100 g (cooked)

Watermelon	0.24 mg per 100 g
Coconut	2.4 mg per 100 g
Sesame seeds	14.6 mg per 100 g
Raisins	4.3 mg per cup
Beets	0.7 mg per cup (cooked)
Beet juice	1.1 mg per cup
Brown rice	1.0 mg per cup (cooked)

While it's not the most iron-rich food, brown rice is still a nutritious choice, offering fiber, magnesium, and B vitamins.

You can also consume iron-fortifying teas, such as stinging nettle, alfalfa root/leaves, dandelion roots/leaves, yellow dock, mint, rosehips, red raspberry, red clover, lemon balm, lemon peel, and lemongrass. For taste and to boost iron absorption, add an herb that has substantial vitamin C, like yellow dock or hibiscus, or add a couple squeezes of citrus, such as a lemon.[4]

TEAS AND HERBS FOR IRON

Note: Some herbs can negatively interact with prescription medications or certain health conditions, so always be sure to talk with your doctor before consuming herbal teas.

Yellow dock tea	While exact values can vary, yellow dock root is considered one of the best plant-based sources of bioavailable iron.
Nettle tea	Known for its iron content, though exact amounts can vary.
Dandelion root tea	Contains approximately 0.5 mg of iron. While it's not the highest source of iron, dandelion root is often used in herbal blends to support iron levels, especially when combined with vitamin C–rich herbs to enhance absorption.
Alfalfa leaves	Naturally rich in iron, calcium, and vitamin C, making the tea a beneficial option for increased iron levels.
Ginger	Helps with nausea, digestion, and the absorption of iron.
Hibiscus tea	Contains 0.71 mg of iron per cup and is rich in vitamin C, making it a great choice for boosting iron intake.
Red raspberry tea	Contains 0.3 mg of iron per cup.
Fresh spearmint leaves	Contains 12 mg of iron per 100 g.

POSTPARTUM IRON HEALING TEA RECIPE

12 cups of water
5 tablespoons fresh ginger
3 tablespoons red raspberry herbs

2 tablespoons yellow dock
2 tablespoons spearmint
Raw organic honey, for taste

You can make this on the stove in a stock or soup pot. Fill the pot halfway with water, bring to a boil for 10 minutes with ginger, then once boiling, turn the fire off and add the rest of the ingredients. Cover and let steep for 15 minutes. Strain the tea, and serve to mama with or without honey. Whenever mama is thirsty and needs a warming, restorative drink, heat up and serve.

Pot Likker

Pot likker, or pot liquor, is the liquid leftover from cooking fish, poultry, meats, tomatoes, and greens with vinegar, historically in a black cast-iron pot (for added iron). This homemade broth alone can provide two to five milligrams of iron. To make it, cook greens down with animal bones and one to two teaspoons of vinegar for about thirty minutes. The older generations cooked their greens for extended periods on a low simmer. This was done because the women knew that the longer the greens and bones cooked, the easier it would be to digest and the more potent the pot liquor medicine would become.

Pot likker is valued as medicine because it contains plenty of vitamins and minerals like vitamins A, B-6, C, D, E, K, folate, niacin, riboflavin, thiamin, potassium, magnesium, iron, calcium, phosphorus, sodium, zinc, and protein—all of which help restore mama and baby's health, strength, and energy. Traditionally, it was consumed in multiple forms, including in gravies, stews, soups, and even as a warm drink. It was never discarded and should not be wasted.

Fermented Foods

Fermented foods are great for the health of our gut microbiome, offering probiotics and prebiotics, which nourish the good bacteria in our stomachs.[5] In addition to balancing this microbiome, fermented foods also help support digestion, reduce inflammation, fortify the immune system, and can make the nutrients in foods more bioavailable.[6] For these reasons, they are great for overall recuperation in the early postpartum period.

A broad range of fermented foods, drinks, and condiments have a long history in African culture, and many have been passed down and adapted for our current African American traditions. A common fermented postpartum food is cornbread soaked in buttermilk and sprinkled with a little sugar. Buttermilk in the South was discovered by enslaved Africans when they found that their leftover milk had fermented at the bottom of the barrel. I grew up watching my dad drink buttermilk, and as a child, I didn't like it at all. As an adult, though, I better appreciate the taste and certainly understand its health benefits.

Buttermilk has a host of benefits for postpartum healing, such as lowering systolic blood pressure; speeding up healing due to its protein, vitamin B-12, riboflavin, enzyme, and mineral content; improving digestion; and promoting relaxation and sleep. After the baby is born, new mothers should drink a glass of room-temperature buttermilk daily to improve their overall postpartum recuperation.[7]

Another traditional fermented condiment is cha-cha (or chow-chow), which is a mixture of shredded cabbage, diced green tomatoes, jalapeño peppers, red peppers, onions, special spices, apple cider vinegar, and cane sugar (or organic honey). Once thoroughly mixed, these ingredients are thermally processed in a large kettle, canned, and left to ferment. I recommend that new mamas add cha-cha to their greens, butter beans, rice, and stews. My grandma always kept plenty of cha-cha in the storage closet, which she canned herself every summer and fall. I always loved the spicy taste.

Besides buttermilk and cha-cha, the Granny Midwives also fed new mothers pickled vegetables and fruits to help improve digestion.[8] Pickled foods may include beets, string beans, carrots, okra, cucumbers, turnips, watermelon rinds, and eggs. These make a wonderful, healthful side with dinner or a warm snack.

Replenish Your Bones

Your baby used your calcium to grow their bones while in the womb, and your uterus used calcium to facilitate labor contractions, so during postpartum you need to replenish your calcium stores for bone and teeth health. Research shows that women who were born and lived in the South during the 1920s had lower rates of osteoporosis; this has been attributed to them regularly consuming potent pot likker, which is full of calcium, vitamins C and K, and potassium—vital nutrients for bone health.[9] Additionally, the Granny Midwife often used cast-iron pots to cook her beans, vegetables, and meat with bones intact. These food combinations help replace lost minerals, including calcium.

My Alabama Granny Midwives also taught me about the bone-strengthening power of sunbathing before birth and late postpartum. A few weeks into the postpartum period, I instruct mamas to sit in the morning sun to warm up and get some vitamin D, which improves their mood and helps their body absorb all the good calcium they're consuming.

Healthy Snacks

New mamas will want good snacks to eat in between meals to support their emotional and physiological well-being. Light snacks are easy to make, consume, and digest. Some healthy nutrient-rich postpartum snacks include sautéed liver, bananas warmed in coconut milk, a cup of warm buttermilk sprinkled with a dash of cinnamon, soft scrambled eggs lightly sprinkled with salt, sautéed deveined shrimp, black-eyed peas, and warmed dried fruit, like prunes, dates, apricots, and figs, sauteed in honey with a dash of cinnamon or nutmeg.

Sweets for Postpartum Happiness

Granny Midwives knew birth was a celebration and a blessing, and thus special desserts were needed during the lying-in to bring a smile to the mother. Some common desserts were deep-dish soupy peach cobblers, buttermilk peach pie, and apples sautéed in butter with sugar and a dash of cinnamon, clove, and nutmeg. African Americans inherited pudding from our African ancestors, turning it into sweet potato, rice, coconut, and banana puddings; these are great for making mamas happy. You can also make buttermilk pie, a classic Southern dessert with a creamy, custard-like filling and a slightly tangy flavor. It's made with buttermilk, eggs, sugar, butter, and vanilla, and it adds additional healthy calories for breastfeeding mothers.

Keep an Eye on Meal Timing

New mothers need two to three delicious, spicy meals per day. "Spicy" means meals that contain warming aromatics and spices, like onions, garlic, rosemary, bay leaves, basil, nutmeg, ginger, chili, cayenne, fennel, cloves, and cinnamon. These spices smell good, can improve appetite and the taste of food, and help with digestion. Many of these spices are also anti-inflammatory and rich in antioxidants, which work to improve health outcomes.[10]

Mamas should always have savory snacks and yummy desserts

on her nightstand to eat between meals. New mothers should consume an extra five hundred calories per day when breastfeeding. The lying-in period is their time to eat well and not restrict calories so they can properly nourish their body and brain. Start by eating three or four small meals and adjust them as needed. Each mama is different; she may eat a lot and require snacks, or it may take her some time to build an appetite. Regardless, a consistent meal schedule will help her get strong, so don't let her go hours without eating. It's also best that she drinks a warm beverage thirty minutes before eating.

Nourish Your Body and Soul

Be mindful of what you consume and where it comes from. Food receives its strength to sustain life from minerals in the soil and the sun's rays, which allow the plants to hold energy at the molecular level and create chlorophyll, which brings health to the human body. Food sprouts from the womb of Mother Earth; it is her medicine to the world. Our job is to honor and protect our health by respecting food and being intentional about what we eat.

The food that goes into your body should be sacred, clean, and nutritious. Some restaurants serve food that is unhealthy and unfit for consumption, which can lead to illnesses, such as diabetes, obesity, cancer, and hypertension. When postpartum mothers are fed fast food and dry foods with empty calories, they will have low energy, poor digestion, constipation, and a weaker immune system.

> *Remember that not all food is medicine, so choose your diet wisely. Use the recipes in this book to make healthy choices for postpartum healing.*

MAKE IT COMMUNAL FOR HIGHER VIBRATIONS

In her 2008 book *Harambee! Stories and Recipes from the African Family Circle*, Kenyan author Grace Kuto says that, in Kenya, cooking food is about bringing family together and staying connected.[11] This is also a core concept in African American culture. Food is not just a source of nutrients but also a means of bringing people together and creating a sense of community and trust. In our culture, food holds a special place in all aspects of life, from happy to solemn occasions. When people are relaxed, eating together, and enjoying one another's company, it raises the community's healing vibration (or, as science would put it, it raises our oxytocin levels). Similarly, African American postpartum traditions use meals to bring the new mama's family together to be a part of her emotional nourishment and reduce postpartum depression.

It may not always be possible for someone to be with you while you eat, but having at least one person eat with you can increase your endorphins and give you a sense of tranquility. Mothers like it when I eat with them or keep them company because many are often home alone when their partner is at work or running errands for the family. If it's not possible to eat with a companion, call a friend and have lunch together over Zoom or put on your favorite comedy show while you eat. You could also play some instrumental music or eat in silence if that makes you happy, but try your best not to eat while watching the news or a suspenseful movie.

In our tradition, it is customary for family members to cook together, like my sisters and husband did for me. Cooking together infuses mama's food with community energy. Think of it like nutritional prayers. You can also pray directly over the food, asking it to work as a source of nourishment for you and your family.

> ### Connected Through Cooking
> In the African American family, cooking is for health and independence, and it is a rite of passage. It is how mothers prepare their children to care for themselves and their families, so they can make the postpartum soups for their daughters, sisters, and wives one day. We "celebrate Black mothers and children who practice cooking as an art form and a demonstration of self-reliance and healing."[12]

SERVING THE MOTHER

It's not just about the food itself, but the way you serve it as well. Serving food properly is another way you can love and honor the mother. The most important part of the postpartum period is reassuring the mother that she is safe, everything is normal, and she is doing an excellent job. Serving the mother warm, delicious food and keeping her company as she eats is a wonderful way to do this. When you make her food, make it with love to heal her because love creates oxytocin, the soothing hormone released during loving activities like hugging and bonding. When you give her food, treat her like a queen because motherhood is the highest status in the world.

Often, a mother will feel weak, sad, and hungry early in her postpartum period because she is unable to prepare food to eat. A new mother who is tired, fatigued, emotional, or irritable could be both hungry and thirsty and not realize it. Offering and serving a new mother excellent quality and tasty foods with a pretty presentation can help her feel beautiful, special, and secure, and a secure mother is more likely to develop her mothering skills and build confidence, principal factors for mental health.

For these reasons, I try not to serve any of a new mother's meals on a paper plate. I prefer to serve her food on a porcelain plate and put a flower on her tray. Make serving her a ceremony. Beautify it and elevate it, even in small ways. Regardless of the economic situation, I make a beautiful presentation using what the family has, or I may bring something from my home to help her feel honored.

Nourishment for Cesarean Births

Mothers who give birth via cesarean section need nourishment that addresses the impact of the surgery. Whether the cesarean was planned or an emergency, the mother's whole being—conscious and subconscious—is impacted by the experience, and she needs reassurance that she did a good job. Often, more blood is lost with this intervention, so new mothers need to be nourished with foods that are high in iron, calcium, and magnesium. She'll also need at least seventy grams of protein per day to help her incision heal, and she'll need plenty of fat-soluble vitamins, such as vitamin A, E, D, and K, as well as foods rich in B vitamins, which play a significant role in supporting postpartum emotional health and aiding brain function.[13] Vitamin C will also help strengthen the immune system.

The good news is African American postpartum foods provide these needed benefits for good postoperative healing. To prevent complications, keep in mind that the mother's body has extra healing to do: her body and psyche are recuperating from having the baby and having surgery. Even when a cesarean section is completed without complication, it is a burden to the body, and nourishment is essential to heal properly, lessen postoperative pain, and avoid infection.

NOURISHED BEYOND FOOD

In the African American postpartum culture, nourishing the mother also means encouraging, supporting, and developing her emotionally. The mother and baby are both sacred and a blessing, and carrying and bringing forth new life is a sacrifice for humankind. The mother must be encouraged and celebrated in this accomplishment.

New mothers and babies need to be engulfed in positive energy. Sad or suspenseful news as well as any and all violence should be avoided by new mothers, infants, and small children. I advise mothers to avoid the news and shut down their phones or assign it to a family member to monitor their calls. Seeing sad and stressful news during the postpartum period can have negative effects on both mother and the baby. Because of our collective historical and daily trauma, African Americans mothers in the United States are at an increased risk for PTSD.[14] As a Black postpartum mother, you need to be cared for with a lot of sensitivity, calming teas, and plenty of massages.

Some symptoms of postpartum PTSD include heightened anxiety, increased sleepiness, frequent headaches, and ongoing digestion problems. If this is the case for you, share your feelings with a trusted person and protect yourself from all negativity, including the news. Listen to positive, uplifting music and watch comedy shows for a mood boost. You can also drink calming herbal teas, such as lemon balm, chamomile, and lavender. And, of course, don't be afraid to seek medical advice as needed. When caring for a Black postpartum mother, nourish her by shielding her from negative people and experiences. It's the community's job to create a protective circle around her and the new baby.

Today, the need to reassure a new mother of her beauty and power is more paramount than ever as we witness the erasure of the word "mother" and the lowering of her status. Birth is emotional, and that is normal, but the new-age mother is bombarded with false narratives from Western philosophy that says your birth defines you. New mothers are currently being distracted by all the noise that focuses on irrelevant data about the birth experience instead of on becoming a mother and indulging in the joy of her newborn.

It's important that you celebrate yourself, regardless of your birth experience. You are not a failure if you departed from your drug-free birth plan and instead requested an epidural or agreed to a cesarean section. This is where the spirituality of birth comes into play. We can do everything according to the books of eating right, being in a loving relationship, staying active during pregnancy, hiring a midwife, and planning a home birth, but birth is an uncontrollable event, and it will humble us. There is an outside force at work, and at the end of the day, it doesn't really matter how our babies get earthside. We must be kind to ourselves, knowing we did the best we could to birth a healthy baby.

So, release yourself of self-doubting questions, like "Did I birth successfully?" "Did I protect my birth plan?" or "Did the medical team respect me?" This anxiety will only follow you into your postpartum period, potentially overshadowing your peaceful time with your newborn. Your lying-in period is a time for you to be with your baby, spouse, partner, family, and birth workers. And our job as your caregivers is to encourage you to tell your birth story, listen without judgment, and reassure you that you did everything right.

In the African American philosophy of having children, motherhood is the most respected position on earth. In our culture, as far back as we can go, having a baby was seen as a blessing, and large families were viewed as spiritual and physical investments. Modern-day Western propaganda has given Black women space to doubt their ability to mother, recuperate through the postpartum experience, and come out on the side whole, happy, and with a healthy baby. With African American nourishment practices, we validate the mother's experiences and acknowledge the postpartum period as a rite of passage. The mother's work to birth new life deserves celebration. She participated in a divine act, so she must be nourished by all those around her. We do not linger on the negative after the baby is born alive. Society likes to pry into how the birth was, and not how the mother and baby are now and how they can help. With our traditions, we turn this prying on its head and call the new mother back to her mother's womb, the place where she was fed, nurtured, nourished, and where she first gained confidence to be born.

NOURISHING MAMA IS NOURISHING BABY

Nourishing the mother with healthy food and community protection contributes to the baby's nourishment and improves the bonding relationship between mother and baby. Food is medicine and critical for full postpartum recuperation. Don't stress about it, but commit to consuming high-quality, nutritious foods using the healthy meals mentioned in this book. It is lifesaving and life-giving.

CHAPTER 7

Hydrated and Healed

We thank the Creator for water. Water is the symbol of many things—renewal, rebirth, and life itself. There is no life without water, and all life comes from it, the water of the womb.[1]

We thank the Creator for herbs that grow with the nourishment of water, sunlight, and soil. We're thankful for their medicine and the way they can lull us to sleep, keep us calm and warm, restore our health, and connect us to the earth and to light.

Let this mother grow strong through water and herbs. Let them heal her, hydrate her, and bring nourishment to all the muscles, tissues, and bones of her body. Make her breastmilk abundant and her mind strong.

OUR POSTPARTUM TRADITIONS COULD NOT EXIST WITHOUT THE use of nature's medicine—herbs and spices—which help bring women's bodies, minds, and spirits back to a state of wellness. Enslaved Africans brought their herbal wisdom with them, and they also learned how to use North American herbs and plants from local Indigenous people and European settlers.[2] Elder women used a variety of methods to administer the herbs and spices needed to help new mothers heal and gain strength. Tonic drinks, like sassafras tea, pine needle tea, citrus tea from orange and lemon peels, and dandelion leaf tea, were fairly common. Granny Midwives would also make cotton root bark tea to prevent abnormal bleeding, or they'd put a dash of cayenne pepper in warm, honey-sweetened water to create heat in the body and help the mother sweat out toxins. They would also rub new mothers with herb-infused oils and flora water to keep their limbs and back strong. Hydration and herbal traditions give mamas a strong start for long-term quality of life, whether they conceive again or not.

As we've previously discussed, labor and birth naturally cause an excess loss of body fluids from crying, urinating, sweating, vomiting, bowel movements, labor breathing, blood loss, and breastfeeding, so it's important that postpartum mothers stay hydrated with warm liquids. This is another reason why Granny Midwives offered the new mother warm soup immediately after birth. It not only worked to nourish her, but it also quenched her thirst and replaced her electrolytes stores. Warm liquids infused with herbs, roots, barks, and plants are powerful hydrating drinks to serve the mother's full-body recuperation.

Herbs and plant medicine also help reduce swelling, increase breastmilk supply, support digestion, balance blood sugar, and encourage restful sleep.

HEALING TONICS AND MEDICINAL FLUIDS

In the early 1900s, herbal tonics played a crucial role in preparing the mother for pregnancy, childbirth, and postpartum care. These tonics were often made from medicinal plants, roots, and herbs that had been passed down through generations.[3]

Blessed Water

There is a strong tradition of infusing water with the energy from rocks, herbs, spices, and salts. Most herbal infusions in the Black postpartum tradition begin with water as it is a universal healer. As you may have already noticed, many of our postpartum healing practices are water based: baths, warm compresses, soups, stews, teas, broths, gravies, etc. Water is powerful, helping to carry nutrients from food to the stomach and eliminate toxins from the body. Research has shown that water is actually alive, and that it is molecularly affected by energetic feelings, vibrations, and intentions.[4]

Water is sacred and cleansing. When I prepare a bath for a new mama, I bless the water that will be used. I thank God for the water and pay homage to its source by remembering the power of the ocean and acknowledging the fact that unborn humans spend roughly the first forty weeks of their lives in water. For this reason, I like to say the following prayer over the water: "Thank you, Creator, for the power of the water, for its two hydrogen atoms and one oxygen atom. I recognize that water is living, and I ask for blessings on this water. Let it be a medicine, a vehicle to dissolve any physical illness, cleanse the mother of inner turmoil, and replace it with peace and relaxation. We wash it away. Amen."

Herbal Infusions, Broths, and Teas

Coconut water is a powerful healing drink with many nutritional benefits for the postpartum period. Though it's already sweet, you can add mint leaves to make it sweeter. Pot likker and bone broth can also be categorized as nutritious infusions. Infusing blessed water with herbs and nutrient-rich foods amplifies their healing properties. Pot likker is a great example of this, as the leftover liquid from cooking fats, greens, beans, and other vegetables is an excellent source of hydration and healing. All mothers, but especially those who feel weak or dehydrated after giving birth, should be given pot likker that had bones cooked in it. You can offer both warm in a cup, or she can drink it like soup from a bowl.

Teas come in many specific formulations to expel gas from the mother, increase her breastmilk supply, relieve a colicky baby, and restore hydration. Teas like red raspberry leaf, alfalfa, nettle, and ginger are great to replenish any lost fluids. Cinnamon, ginger, and black pepper tea can be given for afterbirth pains. Dandelion root and chicory root tea are good purgative teas to help clean out the mother's bowels (Granny Midwives also gave a tablespoon of castor oil to relieve constipation). Catnip, chamomile, lemon balm, red clover, and mint teas can help reduce anxiety and improve sleep quality. A gentle sleepy-time tea infusion consists of one teaspoon each of chamomile, lemon balm, and mint to two cups of water. Or for a stronger infusion, one teaspoon each of hops and valerian root. This option tastes bitter, and honestly, some mamas don't like it, but it certainly works! If the taste is too unbearable, you can give the mother a teaspoon of raw honey afterward. As always, check with your healthcare provider to make sure you are okay to consume certain herbs.

You'll find lots of recipes for hydrating teas and infusions in chapter 10, including wassail tea, which is made with orange, pineapple, and apple juice as well as whole cinnamon and cloves; catnip and cinnamon bark tea infused with raspberry, ginger, alfalfa, and nettle; fennel and peppermint tea; tender coconut water, which helps reduce swelling in the hands and feet, support digestion, and relieve constipation; and fennel seed, nettle leaf, blessed thistle, and vervain tea for increased breastmilk supply.

Tea Ritual

One thing I like about the era of the Granny Midwives is their wisdom of taking it slow, not rushing, keeping faith in their caregiving work, and believing that God was guiding them in their actions. They used teatime for what it had been for centuries: a time to socialize, build community, relax, recharge, and enjoy the moment.

When I visit new mothers, I like to bring a cup of tea for her and me so I can sit with her for a moment. Sharing a cup of tea rather than a meal prevents me from sitting too long and tiring her out with over-socializing. To keep her satisfied but not too full, give her tea in an eight-ounce teacup. This smaller amount also encourages her to savor the drink. Teatime with mama fulfills multiple purposes: It is a way to ensure that she's well-hydrated, it gives you as the caretaker a chance to sit and enjoy her company, and it is a great opportunity to connect with the mama and hear how she is doing and what she wants and needs. You can also observe how the baby is doing with the mama and on their own.

Teatime is an excellent opportunity to naturally observe how mama is coping in her postpartum period. Is she falling asleep while holding her cup of tea? If so, gently take the cup from her hand and let her sleep. You can always rewarm it on the stove when she wakes up. Let it remain at room temperature and cover it with a saucer.

When drinking tea with mama, listen to her words. Is she saying that she is exhausted or can't cope? If so, explore the cause and see how you can find ways to support her. When a mother says she is feeling exhausted, that is a warning sign of a setback.

A "setback" is when a new mother takes on too much too soon and gets sick during her lying-in period. Things that cause a setback include doing housework, leaving the house too often, cooking, walking the dog, or driving children to school—basically any activities that interrupt her forty-two days of postpartum rest. Other signs of a setback include going from a light flow back to heavier bleeding, or from a pink bleed back to red bleeding; body aches, particularly lower back, pelvic, and incision pain; headaches, exhaustion, frequent crying, and melancholy. The goal is to help prevent a setback at all costs, and this is done by reassuring the mother, listening to her concerns, validating her reality, letting her know that you are there to support her, and reminding her to keep her feet elevated and avoid picking up anything heavier than her baby.

Teatime or snack time with mama also allows me to rest my body and mind while mama rests. When I bring her a cup of postpartum tea made of red raspberry leaves, nettle, ginger root, and mint with honey, I take a cup for myself and add a bag of caffeinated black tea to give me the extra energy I need. African American postpartum care is not about burning out the caregiver; it is about giving and receiving in equal measure. Those who do this loving postpartum care work must also take care of themselves with teatime and self-care.

HERBAL HEALING FOR POSTPARTUM DISCOMFORTS

The US medical system has normalized many postpartum discomforts as unavoidable, but the Granny Midwife had a cure for most of them. Though certain uncomfortable things do result from birth, using African American postpartum traditions can often offer immediate relief or shorten the timeline of discomfort. For example, a sore vulva, engorged breasts, and fatigue are all normal, but mothers do not need to suffer with these for their entire postpartum period. In most cases, these symptoms can be managed and shortened using the traditions of our ancestors, like postpartum baths, warm herbal compresses, and hydration for healing. We have many ways to use herbs for postpartum healing.

Vulva Pain or Burning

Because of the natural stretching of the vulva for baby's birth, or due to an episiotomy, soreness and a burning sensation can be expected with the first few urinations after birth. This can also be the case if the mother needed a catheter during her labor and birth. To assist in healing and bringing immediate comfort, use warm compresses saturated with a warm comfrey decoction as soon as the placenta is delivered.[5] Once the compress is cooled, re-submerge it in a pot of very warm comfrey decoction and reapply. Repeat this five to ten times. Then, wash the vulva with a warm tea of comfrey, ginger, and sage water on day one only. Thereafter, continue with this vaginal wash, minus the sage, for four weeks.

I like adding comfrey (*Symphytum officinale*) because, traditionally, it is used for wound healing, joint pain relief, and inflammation reduction. It contains a compound called allantoin that promotes cell regeneration, making it popular for treating bruises, sprains, and muscle injuries.[6] I love the comfrey plant as a postpartum herb because when I tore with my second birth, I sat in the herb almost daily for four weeks and had amazing results. Please note that, according to the FDA, comfrey should only be used externally and not consumed orally.

Tips for Using Comfrey

There are several ways to use comfrey for vulva and perineum healing.

Basic preparation: Boil two cups of water, turn the water off, and add a half cup of dried comfrey leaves. Cover the pot and let it steep for fifteen minutes. Strain the tea, then use it as you wish. You can fill a twenty-four-ounce plastic pitcher with warm comfrey tea and pour it over the vulva while the mother is urinating to dilute her urine, begin healing any sore areas, and minimize the burning sensation. Repeat this for the first twenty-four hours after birth or until the stinging stops. You can also mix comfrey tea with rosemary and ginger for a sitz bath.

Once the burning sensation has passed, you can put the comfrey tea in mama's postpartum peri bottle to help heal the vulva area. It can take anywhere from six to twelve weeks for the vulva to heal completely. You can also place warm comfrey compresses over the vulva and/or add the same comfrey formula to a sitz bath every day for ten days, then every other day until day twenty, then a few times a week until the area feels fine. See your healthcare provider if you're not feeling better by the end of your lying-in period.

A few more considerations for vulva and perineum healing:

- During the first forty days, mamas should sit on their side and not directly on the buttocks. This keeps pressure off the vaginal area, prevents soreness, and facilitates healing.
- New mamas can begin very gentle Kegel exercises on day one. It will feel difficult, but it will improve as the weeks go by. Doing Kegel exercises increases blood flow to the vagina and anal area, facilitating healing.

Exhaustion

In our tradition of mothering the mother, we do our best to take exquisite care of the mother so she doesn't exhaust herself from lack of rest, worry, poor sleep, hunger, or isolation. Drinking plenty of liquids and staying hydrated is one way we prevent exhaustion.

To keep her energy levels up, add one teaspoon each of red raspberry leaf, alfalfa, nettle, and ginger and two teaspoons of Gotu Kola to two cups of boiled water, and have mama sip on it throughout the day. Gotu Kola is a perennial herb, often sold in powdered form, that can help with mood, energy, and healing. I prefer using the leaf in my homemade herbal drinks. Other traditions and rituals that are helpful for preventing exhaustion include serving nutritious, warm, iron-rich meals like chicken soup with rice or kale stew cooked with black-eyed peas; providing regular massages in a warm room after showering; dressing mama and putting clean sheets on the bed; drawing the curtains or giving her an eye mask so she can sleep; playing instrumental music for her; and spending quality time with her.

Concerning Signs of Postpartum Exhaustion:

- Looking exhausted
- Saying she is exhausted
- Headaches
- Digestive issues
- Irritability
- Frequent crying
- Sleep issues
- Restlessness
- Sleeping while sitting up
- Perceiving her baby as difficult[7]

If, as a new mother, you feel any of these symptoms, or if you are caring for a mama who is exhibiting them, be sure to strictly follow the postpartum traditions so you can rest, eat, hydrate, and heal.

Postpartum fatigue is not inevitable or universal, although early in the postnatal period, it affects a substantial proportion of women. Predictors include age and parity, but practical help and support from partners and midwives may be protective factors.

Hemorrhoids

Pushing a baby out can create hemorrhoids or push current hemorrhoids out, making the area painful and sometimes itchy. To remedy this, you can place homemade witch hazel pads (witch-hazel-soaked cotton balls) or warmed black tea bags directly on the hemorrhoids. Let them sit for fifteen minutes five times a day. Once the hemorrhoids shrink, try to reinsert them back in the anus, using clean hands and shea butter. Also be sure to place your feet on a stool when having a bowel movement to prevent straining.

Constipation

If you're having trouble making bowel movements, prioritize hydration: Drink eight cups of water daily, plus postpartum soups, broths, and warmed prune juice. You can also do Kegel exercises or walk around the house for five minutes to expel gas. Relax and don't fear the elimination process; it should be painless. Granny Midwives often gave postpartum mothers a tablespoon of castor oil if they had not gone to the bathroom by day three.

Lochia

Lochia is the natural vaginal discharge that occurs for about four to six weeks after giving birth. Using your peri bottle, rinse your vagina with the same healing tea of comfrey, red raspberry leaf, and rosemary before putting on a fresh pad. Change the pad frequently, wear breathable cotton underwear, and by all means, do not use tampons. If you have questions about the color, consistency, amount, or odor of your lochia, call your healthcare provider right away.

Involution

Involution is the shrinking of the uterus, and it is sometimes painful for second-time mothers because they can feel their uterus getting smaller and returning to its original place. Involution is typically brought on by breastfeeding and helps prevent hemorrhaging. To manage the pain naturally, Granny Midwives would have mamas drink ginger and red clover tea. You can also use a hot water bottle, warm rice socks, belly wrapping, and slow labor breathing to ease any pain or discomfort. Involution pain lasts about three to five days, with each day lessening in intensity. If the pain is intolerable, your medical provider can provide ibuprofen.

Engorged Breasts

Congratulations, mama, your milk is coming in! Engorged breasts typically happen on day three, by which time your breasts may look larger and feel heavier, or they may feel lumpy and hard to the touch. The main solution to ease any discomfort is to nurse the baby to get the milk out. You can also hand express, use a breast pump, or take a hot shower and let water run over your breasts as you massage them and get the milk to leak. Alternatively, your partner can suck the milk out as well. If the weight of your breasts is causing issues, you can wrap them with a cotton cloth and hold them up for immediate relief.

Granny Midwives would recommended breastfeeding as the first form of relief. Second would be having your partner suck the milk out, and third would be placing your breast in a bowl of warm water or showering with hot water to help them soften and leak. Use the breast pump as a last resort, only if the previous recommendations are not helping. Engorgement should begin to subside by after two or three days. First-time moms will likely have it more than mothers who have birthed before. For additional relief, you can also drink one to two cups of sage, peppermint, parsley, or sorrel tea on day one and two. Discontinue this after forty-eight hours, unless you plan to dry your milk up. With patience, you will get relief, and your breasts will soften again. Enjoy the journey.

Note: Sore nipples are not engorgement. If you experience sore nipples, check the baby's latch and put a bit of breastmilk on your nipples and air-dry them as a way to heal. To avoid nipple damage and pain, gently help your baby break their suction when taking them off the breast. Ask your lactation counselor to show you how. Whenever possible, keep your nipple exposed to the air, as this helps avoid cracked nipples, and seek support as needed from a lactation consultant.

Body Aches

Postpartum baths infused with ginger, comfrey, and mint leaves, as well as a massage with arnica oil, can help relieve body aches. A poultice from herbs, clay, or other natural ingredients can be applied to the skin to draw out toxins, reduce inflammation, or promote healing. You can put it directly on the sore area or wrap the paste in a thin cotton cheesecloth, and apply it with heat, such as a hot water bottle or rice socks, to alleviate aches. Some women experience jaw aches from clenching their teeth during the pushing phase. If this is the case for you, performing jaw massages and placing warm cloths on the jaw and face can provide relief.

Emotional and Teary

Baby blues are hormonal and normal, typically happening between five and eight days after birth and usually lasting two to five days once it starts. If or when this happens, reassure mama that it is the baby blues and it will pass soon. Red clover, lemon balm, and catnip teas can help regulate her hormones. And a little Gotu Kola and mint tea and sweet potato pie will cheer her up.

Baby blues happen, and it is different from postpartum depression. More serious signs of depression will include mama not feeling like herself, being afraid to be alone with baby, and speaking of not wanting to live. In these cases, immediately call her healthcare provider or drive her to the nearest emergency hospital.

Sweating

Once pregnancy ends, the body immediately begins to expel the water that is no longer needed through increased perspiration. Be sure to keep mama well hydrated, salt her food to taste, encourage her to take frequent showers, and change her bed sheets regularly. As we've discussed, night sweats can last from two to six weeks, before hormones finally balance out.[8]

One easy way to make sure you are getting enough hydration is to keep a pitcher of water near your bed with a favorite mug or crystal glass and empty it twice daily.

CHAPTER 8

Rested

Mama, let your body rest. Let the busyness of the world go on around you while you dream, sleep, and put your feet up. Let it all pass you by during this sacred time of healing and closeness with your newborn. You've worked so hard to create new life, and now it is time to love on your baby and listen to your body's need for sleep and rest. You will be tired, but let it be an invitation to slow down. Feel the support of the bed or couch beneath you as it holds you, calls to you. You deserve to unwind and be refreshed. For in rest, we find that our bodies can repair, our hormones can balance, and our emotions can settle. We come back home to ourselves after walking through this birthing portal.

MANY AFRICAN AMERICAN WOMEN STRUGGLE WITH GETTING enough rest. We come from a legacy of enslavement, where rest was not allowed and the workdays were abusively long. Although these kinds of working conditions are no longer part of our reality, their epigenetic impact still influences our current habits, and society continues to pressure us to work hard, making us feel like we are being lazy if we say we are tired or sleepy. We now live in a society where most of us work hard, long hours throughout our entire pregnancies, leaving us sleep deprived. But I want you to know that you deserve rest and sleep.

Rest and sleep were central to our precolonial postpartum traditions. And history tells us that even during enslavement, our people tried to protect new mothers by offering to do their work so they could get one to two days of rest after birthing their babies. This history is important to know, especially if you feel uncomfortable resting during your postpartum period. Our mothers may tell us that they were up on day three, but we are reclaiming our cultural tradition of being in bed on day three. We must commit to resting and sleeping for healing because these actions are a blessing. We must humble ourselves and embrace these gifts from the Creator. A rested body has the best chance of returning to a state of wellness.

The Granny Midwives knew that exhaustion creates a spiral of maternal illness, including postpartum depression, so they prioritized rest above all else. Women who are well rested after birth tend to recover quicker, and that is important for so many reasons, including improved bonding, breastfeeding, and ability to care for herself and her baby; reduced morbidity; and better lifelong health. Sleep is vitally important for both physical and emotional healing after giving birth. While forgetfulness and brain fog are normal postpartum symptoms, sleep deprivation interrupts the brain from bonding with baby and exacerbates mental health issues, such as anxiety, depression, irritability, crying spells, mood swings, indecision, and executive dysfunction. Exhaustion can also manifest as physical symptoms, like headaches, nausea, vomiting, and gastrointestinal problems, which can all have an effect on our postpartum hormones, such as cortisol, estrogen, prolactin, and thyroid hormones.

Getting quality sleep allows a new mother to better regulate her emotions, which normally fluctuate with her hormones throughout the day. Along with better postpartum recuperation, mothers who rest often and get quality sleep are better able to manage their stress and pain, make it through the day with a good mood, and breastfeed successfully.

Sleep is a physiological gift. It is medicinal and spiritual, putting the body in a regenerative state that allows it to produce growth hormones and repair muscles, bones, and tissues.[1] It also reduces inflammation and strengthens the immune system, which speeds up healing. In the African American culture, postpartum sleep is a ritual that takes mothers from feeling weak and exhausted to strong and energetic so they can care for themselves and their newborn baby with more ease.

Twenty-first-century African American postpartum traditions were strict when it came to rest. The main directive was for new mothers to stay in bed for days and not leave the house for weeks. The "lying-in" was so called because it was a time of rest, of literally lying in bed. That's why it was so crucial that new mothers established a strong support system of family and close friends to cook and feed the household; keep the house clean; and diaper, bathe, and massage the baby. In some traditions, the grandmother would co-sleep with the baby and bring them to the mother only when they needed to be nursed. This allowed the mother to get enough deep sleep without being disturbed.

Today's lying-in allows for more within-the-house movement after the first fourteen days, during which new mothers should remain primarily in bed other than to walk to the bathroom for postpartum showers and baths. I remember on day five of one of my postpartum experiences, I sat in my kitchen with my butt on a pillow, another pillow behind my back, my feet propped up on another chair, resting on a pillow, with a blanket over my knees and a warm cup of tea in my hand. My baby slept in my room with the door open so I could hear her if she woke up or cried. My sisters set me up like this so I could keep them company while they prepared food for me and cleaned my kitchen. When I grew tired, they whisked me off to bed to rest. The Granny Midwives would never have allowed a mother to be in the kitchen because they wanted to avoid setbacks at all costs, but today, we offer mothers a little more flexibility.

It can be challenging to get the sleep and rest you need post-partum. You may need some help getting settled, and you'll likely need to develop a mindset of rest. Research has shown that women who get sleep while the baby sleeps and have enough support to maintain a schedule of six to seven hours of sleep a night recover faster and better than women without help who become more sleep deprived over time.[2]

NORMALIZING POSTPARTUM TIREDNESS

As I mentioned earlier, feeling tired immediately after birth is normal. The first thing I usually hear after the birth of a baby is, "I'm hungry," followed by "I am so tired"—and there are a multitude of reasons for this. Mama may have become sleep deprived in the last trimester of her pregnancy, had a long labor, and lacked nourishment during labor due to hospital policy. This is why having a postpartum soup ready for after birth will jump-start healing and give mama energy to bond with her baby. After she has nursed and bonded with the baby and eaten her postpartum soup, the next course of action is getting some restorative sleep.

It's so important to have realistic expectations regarding fatigue. It is normal to feel tired from birth until twenty-four weeks postpartum. Your body has worked harder than it ever has in order to bring forth life. You are not only tired from your uterus contract-ing with the powerful force to open a tightly closed cervix to ten centimeters while rotating and descending the baby through the vagina, but you also spent the last thirty-eight to forty-two weeks growing a roughly seven-pound baby, two-pound placenta, and one pound of amniotic fluid, as well as an increased blood volume. You should expect to feel tired, even with a good diet and help, because it takes lots of energy to restore the body to its nonpregnancy state. No matter if it is your first birth or your ninth, the cycle of having a baby puts a strain on the body and mind, and these resources can only be replenished with adequate rest. New mothers can benefit from learning the role of sleep in healing, how to get help to implement quality sleep, and what the signs of exhaustion and sleep deprivation look like—lethargy, crankiness, crying, difficulty making decisions, and sadness.

Although natural, pregnancy is a burden on the female body. You enter labor with a normal amount of fatigue from the third trimester, followed by birth and then immediately caring for your newborn. Feeling tired is the body's way of telling you to sleep and begin the healing process. Pregnancy and birth use an enormous amount of energy, so do not underestimate the amount of rest you need to rejuvenate and heal your body and mind. Whenever possible, submit to the fatigue and go to sleep instead of trying to clean, cook, entertain, or scroll on social media. You feel sleepy because your body wants to heal. This is normal and a sign that your body is trying to take care of itself. Practice trusting your body and obeying this message.

THE DIFFERENCE BETWEEN REST AND SLEEP

Rest and sleep are both important, but they are not the same. Sleep is true medicine while rest supports good sleep. Rest is defined as putting the mind and body in a meditative state, meaning not doing anything physical and letting the mind and body relax. Rest is a protective mechanism that allows the mother to give her undivided attention to her newborn and heals the body from stress and fear, which can put unnecessary wear and tear on the hormonal, nervous, and immune systems. Sleep, on the other hand, is a normal physiological function like hunger and breathing. As a result, the benefits of sleep are lifesaving because during sleep, the body enters a state of unconsciousness and inactivity to reset. The latest research confirms that the body does most of its healing when sleeping.[3] Rest alone is not enough, but rest can help you sleep better because it allows your body time to calm down and unwind. While sleep is a normal function of the body, I find that many mothers need support learning how to rest and set themselves up for good, productive sleep.

How to Rest

During my childhood summers in Alabama, everyone rested at the hottest time of the day, which was when the sun reached its highest point in the sky. As children, we often sat on a blanket under the shade of a big tree and were ordered to play quietly, relax, and stay out of the sun. I remember lying on the blanket or talking to the other children while some of us dozed off. In some parts of the world, this is called a siesta. I admit that, despite this experience in my childhood, in my young adult years, I stayed on the go and did not have structured rest. After talking to the Granny Midwives, I learned why rest was important and how to rest.

Like me, many of the mothers I've cared for have to learn how to rest, and in my work, I often show new mothers this skill. So many of us have been multitasking our entire lives, with demanding jobs, businesses, homeschooling, and more, and we do not see rest as a necessity nor do we have any idea how to fit it into our lives. The truth is we have to be intentional about it.

I let mamas know that they can rest by sitting in a quiet place and letting their thoughts wander, reading a book, or aimlessly flipping through a fun magazine. You can even lay in bed and look at your beautiful baby lying next to you. Research states that when a mother holds her baby skin to skin for at least sixty minutes, she achieves a form of relaxation due to the secretion of hormones like oxytocin, prolactin, and endorphins, which all create feelings of tranquility and safety.[4]

New mothers can also rest by reclining on the couch or bed, sipping tea, looking out the window, or listening to music. Rest is any activity that allows your body and mind to be in a state of neutrality, not thinking or worrying about anything, just closing your eyes, elevating your feet, and letting go of all worries. Make sure you rest for about five to fifteen minutes several times a day during the entire lying-in period, and make it a habit to have your back and legs supported and elevated as you rest. Sleeping, catnapping, and dozing off are also welcome and will allow your body and mind to rejuvenate from pregnancy, labor, and birth. Scrolling on your phone is not resting.

Immediately Postpartum

The African American postpartum rest protocol begins on the day of the birth. On day one, help mama walk to the shower so you can evaluate her status. Is she too weak or dizzy to walk? This tradition of walking to the shower helps get her circulation moving for healing and allows blood clots to be expelled, which is important for the uterus to stay firm. Once the shower is complete, put the new mother back to bed so she can get some sleep. While the Granny Midwives generally wanted mothers to rest for forty days straight, they allowed some normal movement, like walking to the bathroom, standing up to have their belly wrapped, and walking to get their baby from a relative, who may have been comforting them while she slept.

GETTING GOOD SLEEP

In a perfect, ideal world, you will sleep after your post-birth meal until you are awakened by your baby, who is either looking for comfort or wants to nurse. Then, after nursing, you will go back to sleep for another two to three hours until your baby needs you again. This is the natural and normal rhythm of caring for a newborn—two to three hours of sleep before waking to feed your baby. You will not become exhausted from this pattern because when you are nursing, your body is prepared for short bursts of deep sleep, knowing that it must wake every few hours either through breastmilk letdown or your sensitivity to your baby's cues. Research shows that breastfeeding mothers tend to get good sleep, even if it is for short durations.[5] The reality is new mothers will not get seven to eight hours of uninterrupted sleep, but if you are able to prioritize good sleep, your body will still heal well and you'll feel good.

The problem with postpartum sleep is not the natural rhythm of short, deep sleep, but the many interruptions and stressors new mothers often face within these short windows of sleep. There can be so many challenges when trying to get good sleep and rest. A hospital birth with a two-day postpartum stay, for example, is often full of interruptions by well-meaning medical staff to check the vital signs of mom and baby. This means that a mother must be awakened from her needed sleep to interact with nurses on shift changes and for standard procedures.

One option to reduce your sleep disturbances is to talk with your doctor or midwife and ask them to space your vital checks if they are stable. In addition, you can reduce time spent on your phone before sleep. The blue light from your device can disrupt your body's melatonin production, which is needed to create the sensation of sleepiness. Using the phone too close to bedtime can increase arousal, making it harder to fall asleep.[6] It's also very easy for you to be bombarded by negative news when scrolling on your phone, and this overt and subconscious worry or fear can create restlessness and insomnia.

So while sleep is a normal physiological function that happens on its own, we often need to be intentional about getting good sleep. Here are some things you and your caregivers can do to help you sleep better:

1. Create a Nurturing Environment for Sleep

Traditionally, the light in mama's room was kept low. The Granny Midwife believed that babies' eyes were not fully developed, and they needed low light to see. Plus, mothers were often overstimulated in bright rooms and were more inclined to get up and start moving around instead of resting. In some communities, the rooms were kept dark for several weeks until the baby's eyes adjusted to the light and to keep the mother's brain sleepy.

As a note to mamas and family members: I know we all want to share pictures of our new baby, but please don't take pictures of the baby using your camera flash, as it does hurt their eyes. You may think the baby is always sleeping and will not open their eyes, but if you draw the curtains or lower the shades, it's almost guaranteed that the baby will open their eyes, confirming that the lights are too bright for them.

In the second trimester, I like to check in with mamas on a few things in preparation for baby's arrival:

- In our modern times, it is a clever idea to purchase blackout curtains to help mother and baby get some sleep. You can also keep an eye mask on hand for mama.
- I always ask mama to show me where she normally sleeps, where she gets the best sleep, and where she spends most of her waking hours. If there is a place in the home where she prefers to sleep and gets better sleep, it's best if that space becomes her postpartum room. Or, if she'd like to sleep in her bedroom but does not usually get good sleep there, we look for a solution. Is the room too hot or too cold? Is it too bright? Is it overlooking the street? Can she smell fumes like car exhaust? Is it too noisy? Is the mattress uncomfortable? All of these concerns should be addressed before birth.

2. Limit Internet Time and Bad News, but Welcome Time with Family and Friends

I recommend that mothers have scheduled internet time, no more than twice a day. And, like the Granny Midwives, I discourage mamas from listening to any bad news. This kind of overstimulation raises cortisol levels and creates anxiety or overthinking, which can lead to restlessness or insomnia. Keeping the postpartum mother off her phone and the internet and away from television is beneficial for her mind, eyes, and body.

Although many in the United States discourage visitors during postpartum, this is not the African American tradition. Interacting with family members who make you feel safe and bring laughter can give you positive stimulation, which can help ease you into a deep sleep. In fact, many mothers have reported that the company of friends and family help them relax, and more relaxation equals less stress, allowing the mother to fall asleep more easily and more soundly. In our culture, it is expected that people will come by to help around the house, which decreases the mother's anxiousness and aids in her ability to rest and sleep.

Limit Screen Time to Increase Rest

Pew Research Foundation says women spend more time on social media than men, depending on the age of the women.[7] This is significant because during the postpartum period, reducing screen time and blue light is needed to get good REM sleep for body regeneration. It will be a challenge, but I encourage you to put your phone down after birth—and even limit the amount of pictures you take of your baby. Perhaps a family member can take photos instead, or you can put a ten-minute timer on your phone so you can resume resting as soon as possible. If you're not intentional, excess screen time can easily limit how much rest and sleep you get, with the long-term effects being feeling tired longer than the six-week postpartum period.

3. Create an Outgoing Greeting with New Baby Information

I highly recommend recording an outgoing greeting that lets people know that the baby was born and any other details you wish to share (date, time, weight, sex, name, etc.). You can then add a few notes on how people can help during this precious time:

- Let them know who to contact (text the aunt, partner, or doula) and that they should share when they can come by to help with specific tasks (watching the toddler, doing laundry, completing other household chores, etc.).
- Let them know if cooked food or groceries are welcome.

4. Remember Your Postpartum Traditions of Massage and Bathing

If the mother cannot sleep due to body aches, first make sure to speak with her healthcare provider. Once the symptoms have been classified as normal postpartum discomforts, it's time to double down on our traditional postpartum remedies. Perhaps the mother needs more sitz baths to soothe her perineum area. Or maybe she could use a massage with warm coconut oil, shea butter, and a drop of frankincense for relaxation and to help her sleep. Along with a massage, serve her a warm cup of chamomile tea mixed with a bit of catnip and lavender to ease her into a deep sleep.

5. Be Willing to Sleep Any Time of Day

You don't have to only sleep at night. Take any opportunity you have to sleep, no matter the time of day. The rule is when the newborn sleeps, the mother should sleep. Ignore the cleaning, cooking, or whatever else you think needs doing, and prioritize your sleep.

Mama Shafia's Twelve Tips for Good Sleep
1. Mother is comfortably full with delicious meals.
2. Mother is well hydrated with water.
3. Mother has emptied her bladder and/or colon.
4. Mother is clean (showered, bathed, etc.).

5. The room temperature is correct for the mother's sleeping.
6. Mother has done mild exercise (stretching, walking around the house, etc.).
7. The bed sheets are clean and fresh, and preferably made with cotton or natural fabrics.
8. The noise level in the home is reduced.
9. Mother has a shoulder-and-back rub/massage to facilitate sleep.
10. Sleep music is on low (instrumental, ocean waves, etc.).
11. Mother drinks a cup of sleepy tea infusion.
12. Mama is reassured that someone will wake her when the baby wakes up. Some mothers are afraid to sleep, believing that they may not hear the baby, so be sure to let her know that someone is on guard to care for the baby while she sleeps.

Your baby thrives by being close to you, so during sleep time, keep the baby in the same room as you. The Granny Midwife would agree, and science says all babies, whether in a crib or bed-sharing, do better when sleeping in the same room as the mother for at least the first six months of life.[8]

Better Infant (and Mother) Sleep

Your newborn will likely sleep better when they are close to you, and many mothers also sleep better when their baby is in the room. One thing you can do to get good sleep with or near your baby is to breastfeed lying on your side with baby facing the breast. This reduces fatigue because you don't have to physically get out of bed.

Another sleep method is to learn how to safely bed-share with the baby. The Granny Midwife encouraged sharing a clean bed, meaning one with simple and sparse bedding. In today's world, there are many ways a baby can be lost, whether it's due to a down comforter, stuffed animals, oversized pillows, or falling out of the bed. Don't worry, though. Bed-sharing can be safe when done correctly by following what's called the "Safe Sleep Seven." If you meet all these criteria, you can safely bed-share with your baby with no worry:[9]

Safe Sleep Seven

1. *Baby must sleep with a nonsmoking parent in a smoke-free household.*
2. *Only sober adults are allowed in the bed with baby (and sober includes no marijuana or medications that cause drowsiness).*
3. *You exclusively breastfeed.*
4. *You have a healthy, full-term baby.*
5. *Baby sleeps on their back, on the inside of the bed, and the bed is pushed against a wall.*
6. *Baby wears light, breathable clothes.*
7. *You have a safe sleep surface, meaning a firm mattress with no extra pillows and blankets.*[10]

If this is something that interests you, talk to your healthcare provider or lactation consultant on how to co-sleep. I slept with all seven of my babies, and it made all the difference for me feeling rested.

CHAPTER 9

Loved

Many believe that God is love and that love is medicine. When you birth your baby, even before the placenta is expelled, you must be greeted with love. You deserve to feel protected, guarded, and held by love as a new mother, regardless of how you birthed your baby into the world.

My wish for you is that you are full of love, for yourself and your baby, and that love fills your home and is a balm for your postpartum healing. I pray that you are safeguarded by a loving community, that you touch and are touched by loving hands, and that you are supported in finding your love of motherhood during these early weeks.

EVERY PRINCIPLE WE'VE DISCUSSED SO FAR IS A PRACTICE OF LOVING the mother, but love deserves its own chapter because it is considered the center of quality postpartum care. Family is sacred across the African continent, and this sentiment has been passed down to us as African Americans and implemented in our postpartum traditions. Thus, love is infused into every aspect of care for the mother and newborn. This love is shown with hands-on care and through the words of our ancestors, like "Praise God!

What a beautiful miracle!" and "I love being a part of this. Thank you, and I love you." Historically, mothers cared for their daughters during the postpartum period, and mothers did it well because they loved their daughter and grandbaby and wanted them both to thrive and blossom. A loving touch, homecooked meals, protective prayers, rituals to keep the mother feeling beautiful, and intentional connection are all ways to love the mother and her newborn.

I often tell postpartum caregivers to care for a new mother the way their mother cared for them when they were ill, or at least the way they wished their mama had cared for them. You must love the mother to give her the energy she needs for her postpartum hormonal health. Her body is constantly working to release oxytocin, the love hormone, and prolactin, which produces breastmilk. Both help to reduce mama's anxiety, and both are best made when the postpartum environment is safe and the mother feels loved and protected.

Nature is perfect and has designed mama to only want to focus on her baby for close to two years. Neuroscience has shown that near the end of the third trimester, a portion of the mother's brain structure changes, physiologically allowing her to focus her attention solely on the baby and understand their coos and body language. This brain rewiring only happens in pregnant females.[1] This is an important evolutionary protection for the baby because if the mother doesn't focus on the baby, they could very easily go without much-needed care, leading to poor development. This miracle of love and connection should be honored, encouraged, and protected. As her family and friends, we support the mother's nature to care and covet her baby, in part by validating that she is in her most God-like state during this period of transformation.[2]

The impact of love during the postpartum period should not

be underestimated but highly elevated. Through the acts of love, the mother is able to reap the benefits of reduced negative energy during the postpartum period, which can help resolve some of her fear and anxiety. Love is protection and builds confidence.

HOW TO PRACTICE LOVING COMMUNITY CARE

I love loving the new mother during her lying-in period, and it shows in all my actions, big and small. For instance, I am strict about making my postpartum visits at the agreed-upon time. I do not want to arrive when mama is sleeping because she needs to get her rest, so I coordinate the best time for me to visit. I remind her to not pick up or clean anything because that is part of my reason for checking on her, to reset her space. I prepare in advance, as if I am attending a sacred rite because I am. I take my ritual bath, put on celebratory attire, gather my postpartum soup and herbs, and bring them with me to the mother's house.

On my way, I focus on why I am going and what I want to accomplish, which is always to bring love, joy, and well-being to mama and her household. I enter her home with an internal prayer and a warm salutation to the house, such as "Peace and blessings, everyone." After entering, I do a second greeting specifically to the mother: "Hey, blessed mother, how are you feeling today?" followed by inquiring about how the baby is doing and how often they are feeding. I do this not only to keep count of her baby's feeding experience, but to track how the mother is engaging with feeding and how much good sleep she is getting. I then offer a hug as a greeting of love. If she is standing when I see her, I hug her right away, but if she is in bed, I wash my hands first, then lean over and hug her, sometimes with one to three motherly kisses on the cheek, as three is my spiritual number and is significant in Islam.

Next, I bring her some soup and take some time to talk with her and listen. I may provide some resources, give her a massage, or offer some humor or prayer. I answer questions when asked, and I offer suggestions gently when I observe that there could be an easier way for mama to find comfort or give the baby relief.

I show love by building her confidence, validating her feelings, and reminding her to surrender to her sacred rites of being a new mother. It does not matter how many children she has; each birth is unique, as she has birthed a new spirit. My goal is to elevate the love in the home and encourage household members to show their love for one another, the mother, and the baby.

Offering prayer, in our best attire, is a part of how we show love. We pray for the babies, mamas, papas, and the entire household. We regularly lay hands on the mother and say, "We love you, so we pray for you." We bring our fussing bag, which has things in it to make the mother feel special, like wrapping cloth for the belly, fragrant anointing oils, clay powders for facials, henna for beautification, hair adornments, beads, ocean shells, ribbons, headbands, journals, plants, and flowers. On every visit, I make a point to fuss over the mother in some way.

I look for ways to offer her loving touch, send her healing energy, and let her know that I care and I am there for her. I may place a hand on her shoulder when I am speaking with her, put a hand on her leg, or even stand at the foot of her bed and gently squeeze the top of each foot. I may even hold her hand for a moment and give it a gentle squeeze.

I also show love to the new mother by explaining to her what she should expect emotionally and physically during her sacred postpartum time. I tell her that this is her dedicated and God-given time to enjoy her baby, rest, and be cared for; that she does not need to move according to any schedule; and that she deserves this care.

I remind her that most mammal mothers are inseparable from their infants, and it is only the human mother that is expected to separate from her infant early.

CREATING A SPACE FOR BIRTH STORIES

As I mentioned before, our society often places a lot of emphasis on birth stories, which I've found can take new mothers out of the joy and ease of the lying-in period. However, I'm also aware that sharing her birth story can be a great form of healing for a new mother. Family members and birth workers should use active listening when the mother shares her birth story as it is necessary that she releases any pent-up emotion from her system. I have had many mothers look at me shamefully and share that they didn't have a good birth because they never made it to the birthing tub and instead squatted to birth their baby. Mothers have also shamefully shared that they asked for an epidural when they really wanted a natural birth. These are all valid reactions that deserve acknowledgment, so it is our job as a community to tell her that her birth experience was not wrong, and she has nothing to be ashamed of.

There is a misguided idea in Western culture that you can control your birth. But in African American culture, we understand that birth is spiritual, and each birth experience is special and needed. When it comes to having a baby, you cannot fail. The postpartum period, among many other things, is a time for acceptance. It's a time of letting go, releasing the need to judge yourself, showing yourself some compassion, and moving on to the next stage of motherhood. This can happen more easily when love is infused in the postpartum period.

If you feel the medical system was negligent during your birth, let me remind you that it is difficult for a woman to birth and fight at the same time, and that you still deserve to love yourself and be loved in your postpartum experience. You can journal or write a complaint to the hospital about your birth experience, share your story with others, read your faith book for guidance, and/or use the Irth App (irthapp.com), which is designed for African American women to share their birth stories. This empowering action can bring some peace to you and your family.

I have seen many mothers who were disappointed with their birth outcome suffer from postpartum depression, which inevitably affected their ability to bond with their baby. The scenarios are numerous. Perhaps you wanted a boy but had a girl, you planned a home birth but ended up in the hospital, you had to have an emergency cesarean section when you wanted a vaginal birth, or maybe you hemorrhaged after birth and are still weak and exhausted due to the loss of blood. Whatever your situation, know that the antidote is a lot of love, a lot of fussing, and ample space to share your birth story without judgment.

Unfortunately, the rate of medical negligence is higher in the African American community due to the social determinants of systemic racism. Therefore, African American women need and deserve a lot of love and compassion during their postpartum experience. These mothers are often healing physically, emotionally, and spiritually, and must process a birth experience that was infused with implicit bias and racism. Systemic racism is an unfair burden to carry, and family members and doulas need to be aware of this so the new mother's feelings and experiences are consistently validated. Often, the partner who witnessed this neglect is an especially important support for helping the mother process what happened, and they too need an outlet. In these instances, counseling for both parents can be important. Call your healthcare provider and ask for an African American therapist, preferably a woman, so mama can openly talk about her birth with someone who understands. You can also get in contact with a Black male therapist for the father or other postpartum support groups.

Sometimes, when I provide care during the forty-two-day lying-in period, the mother will share her birth trauma at every visit, and I've even had mothers who shared their traumatic birth experience with me years later. The emotional and mental anguish that can result from birth must be supported with love and patience during the postpartum period. It takes time to process a traumatic birth experience, and I have found that the best help is to be sympathetic, love the mother unconditionally, and provide her with a safe space to share her feelings and help her rest. Nourish her properly with healthy soups, keep her warm, remind her to love herself unconditionally, and encourage her to release any self-blame.

LOVE AND SPIRITUALITY

In our tradition, healing is spiritual. It comes from the Creator, and it is supported by natural healing tools, like love, prayer, touch, rest, and natural foods. Descended from spiritual people, most African Americans believe there's a higher power, and that we must do what we can do, and then surrender and let God take over. This is not a sign of weakness or giving up; this is our power that comes from having a spiritual connection with the Creator and having faith that we are divinely guided, truly blessed, and living our success right now. The postpartum time is a journey, a blessing, and a challenge, and any woman with the correct support will triumph. In this slow process of healing, there is space for celebration of the new mother and baby, and giving them love through intentional action is one of the ultimate gifts.

Healing Through Baby Love

The idea that the mother must continuously hold her baby to be considered a good mother or establish a strong milk supply is not in line with African American postpartum culture. Family members are fully expected to help with infant care, which includes holding the baby between feedings so mama can eat, sleep, go to the bathroom, take a bath, or walk through the house. It is also culturally appropriate for someone besides the mother to change, bathe, and dress the baby, so mama can rest.

In our tradition, we also allow the mother space to love all over her new baby because this is a part of healing. The postpartum period is not only about helping her body return to its nonpregnant state; it is also about encouraging her to love this miracle called a baby. This is about keeping her in a supportive love bubble with her baby, so she can learn her baby and her baby can learn her.

There are numerous emotional and physical benefits that a mother gets from loving her baby. First, there is a symbiotic exchange of pheromones that creates well-being for both the infant and mama. By holding her baby, she warms them and reminds their body to breathe. Holding her baby also kick-starts uterine contractions to reduce excess bleeding and keeps her breastmilk letdown consistent to aid in the baby's weight gain and health. When a baby's tiny hands knead on the breast, it acts as a natural breast massage, moving milk into the ducts and keeping the breast tissue healthy. When the baby does the breast crawl, their little feet push on the mother's fundus, which also causes the uterus to contract, helping reduce maternal blood loss. In all these ways, mama and baby have a powerful physiological and emotional connection of love that is healing to them both.

PRACTICING SELF-LOVE

Though the mother is thoroughly loved by family, friends, and community during her postpartum period, she can and should practice self-love as well, which can include self-hugs, positive self-talk, and affirmations about her beauty, good health, positive mothering, healthy baby, or anything else she wants to affirm. Caregivers and family can remind mama to love herself and tell her that she deserves the best, including rest and breaks from holding the baby.

Encourage mama to use her postpartum baths as an emotional recharge and not solely as a medicinal act. Soft music in the bathroom, low lights, and the smell of lavender flowers and rosemary twigs are all a form of self-care that can remind the mother to relax, slow down, engage in full-belly breathing, enjoy the herbal aromas, and think positive thoughts as she lets her shoulders soften in the heat of the bath.

I also recommend that mothers give themselves a breast massage during their baths. To do this, make sure your hands are warmed by the medicinal water, then massage your breast toward the nipple to reduce engorged breasts and mastitis. As you do so, thank the Creator for your miraculous body that produces perfect milk for your baby. Or you can put warm olive oil on your hands, and starting from the top of your collar bones, gently massage all the way down to your beautiful, darkened areolas. Then, do the same movement starting from the top of your armpit, down to the areola, and over the nipple. Place a hand under your breast and rub upward to the areola. Then, finally, take both your hands, and starting from between your breasts, rub toward the sides of your breast. I encourage you to hold your breast with the hand on the same side and use the opposite hand to massage your breast and see if you can squeeze any milk out.

This quick self-massage is a wonderful way to show love to your breasts, create a loving relationship with them, prevent mastitis, and practice manual expression. If you weren't able to express milk right away, it will become easier as you become more familiar with your breasts and the technique. Along with the relaxing massage, this exercise is also a self-healing technique and a continuation of a self-breast exam, where you become familiar with which lumps are normal for your breasts and which need to be accessed by your healthcare provider. Breast self-exams should continue after the baby is weaned to detect any abnormalities before they become a problem, and they should be practiced during menopause as well.

Self-love is a commitment to African American postpartum traditions and rituals, and another way you can practice it is with daily affirmations. They can be about anything you want to celebrate or honor yourself for. Here are a few examples:

- I am beautiful.
- I am loved.
- I live in abundance.
- I am rested.
- I am being helped.

Along with affirmations, you can make commitments to yourself to practice daily self-care, such as:

- I will eat ninety grams of protein per day.
- I will drink three cups of red raspberry, ginger, nettle, and mint tea.
- I will sleep when the baby sleeps.
- I will rest often with my feet up.
- I will eat when I am hungry.

- I will schedule internet time twice a day for ten minutes.
- I will ask for and accept help.
- I will drink at least thirty-two ounces or more of water a day.
- I will consume an additional 450–500 calories per day when breastfeeding.
- I will stay in a positive environment of love, laughter, and hugs.
- I will get daily sunshine.
- I will keep my baby near me to reduce stress.
- I will do gentle movements and stretches.
- I will breathe deep from my belly.
- I will only pick up the weight of my baby.

Loving yourself also means embracing your body's changes, and if insecurities arise, remember your beauty and power. There are so many advantages to these physical changes. For instance, when you breastfeed for at least twelve months, you reduce your risk of breast cancer and cervical cancer. Breastfeeding can also heal anemia by delaying your menses and prevent diabetes for up to ten years if you're prone to it.[3] So, yes, your breasts might have changed, but now you are living a longer, healthier life, and your baby is healthier in the process. Breastfeeding is beautiful, and the new shape of your body is too. Love this change and embrace the beauty of being a mother, aka a "life giver."

LOVING FAMILIES

Postpartum care is a collective endeavor. The extended family must encourage the dad to be an active participant in the care of the mother. The baby is connected to both the mother and father, for they carry DNA from each parent. Though the mother carries and births the baby, the father is physiologically connected to her through the baby, and thus also has a role in healing himself and her. If there is discord in the house, there can be no positive postpartum healing. This is especially true if there are unresolved issues between the mother and father or the mother and her mother. Any tension will negatively impact the mother's postpartum recuperation, so this has to be dealt with right away.

I always remind fathers and partners that patience is fundamental. During pregnancy, labor and birth, and the postpartum period, mama is experiencing so many things in her mind and body, including a profound love for the new baby, a flood of hormones that mandate bonding and nesting, physical discomfort, fatigue, and some physical and emotional things that do not have words. When I enter a home, I take time to speak with the couple on the importance of being kind to each other and sharing their feelings using "I statements." I congratulate the father for having a new baby and remind him or educate him on how important his role is to nurture, provide, and protect the mother and baby until the mama feels stronger and well. That can take anywhere from three to twelve months. Each mother is different in how they will recuperate, and it has a lot to do with her health prior to pregnancy, the type of labor and birth she had, and the amount of love that is present in her postpartum environment.

I also explain to the father what is happening with the baby, who needs to be breastfed and near mama, and how he too needs time to bond with and warm the baby by holding them close. I tell him that if the mother does not observe the traditions of the lying-in period, she puts herself at risk for maternal depression, illness, and even death. I share all of her needs for the next forty-two days, including her meals, assistance with household chores, and complete abstinence until after the forty-two days. I tell the dad to show the mother affection with touch, tell her how beautiful she is, ask if she needs anything, and use his intuition to bring her things without her having to ask.

Of course, fathers have needs too, and the Granny Midwife was sensitive to that. She made sure to encourage them and listen to them. When I make a home visit, I encourage mama and dad to have some alone time together, offering to hold the baby in another room if they are awake. They often decline because they want to keep the baby with them, and sometimes even their toddlers. I celebrate the blessed role of the father. I remind the mother that the father needs her love and kindness as well, and I encourage them to enjoy nonsexual intimacy.

Loving Through Conflict

When I meet fathers who tell me they are separated or estranged from the mother, I ask them how they plan to support their baby so their child doesn't suffer from failure to thrive syndrome. How will they protect them from illness, or even death? When they say they are not sure, I tell them about the postpartum medicine called "love." I explain how showing love to the mom in the form of respect and compassion will translate to the health of his infant. I encourage fathers to show their baby's mother unconditional love for the sake of their baby's well-being.

Some examples of things single papas can do when they are separate from the mother include sending groceries or cooked meals to the house, covering the cost of a postpartum doula or cleaning service, encouraging his family members to help on his *behalf, or sending flowers or cards with cash or gift cards. I often explain to fathers that a physically and emotionally healthy mother is the best medicine for his new infant, and when he is compassionate to the mother, he sends love to his infant as well. Fathers should always find a way to help the postpartum mother of their infant, regardless of the circumstances, because at some point, visitation will be established, even if it is in adulthood, and every father wants to let their child know that they were loved and cared for, even when they were denied visitation. This will show the child that they were always loved.*[4]

LOVING MOTHERHOOD

Loving what we do and who we are is medicine; therefore, loving motherhood and our mothers is good for us. I recognize that not every pregnancy resulted from an act of love nor were they all desired. In those situations, the community surrounds the mother with love to help her bond with her baby and herself as a mother. The majority of Black people see motherhood as a blessing from God, and Black women often see motherhood as a source of strength, resilience, and cultural pride. We acknowledge that the legacy of anti-Blackness caused Black mothers undue hardship, making the situation more difficult than it should be. And "still we rise," as Maya Angelou wrote.

Historical judgments on Black mothers include myths that we are neglectful mothers, overly strict, and that the fathers of our children are absent. These are myths that can impact how Black mothers receive postpartum care and how they care for themselves during the postpartum period. And, of course, there are similar myths about Black fathers as well, but according to the CDC, Black fathers are 70 percent more active in caring for their children compared to white and Hispanic fathers.[5] Black fathers have higher rates of bathing, diapering, dressing, and helping toddlers use the toilet on a daily basis.

As a new mother, be easy on yourself. Just because you do not feel immediately bonded to your baby after birth does not mean you do not love your baby. Approximately 20 percent of mothers do not bond with their baby at birth or within the so-called "golden hour," the first hour after baby is born, when skin-to-skin contact and bonding are considered especially important.[6] One reason for the forty-two-day lying-in period is to have the quiet time to intuitively create a relationship with your baby, learn who you are, get to know your baby's personality, and discover how you want to mother.

The main difference we've run into in modern times is that we no longer have Granny Midwives and other elder women to teach us about motherhood in the last trimester of pregnancy. Knowing what to expect helped new mothers embrace the love of motherhood. Hearing the challenges and benefits of motherhood as they learned how to sew baby clothes, practiced bathing and diapering someone else's baby, and made diapers to empower themselves as new mothers to know what to expect. This, along with other information, offered new mothers confidence, so when their baby was born, they knew how they might feel, how to hold the baby, and how to care for them properly.

When you are told how special you are as a mother and are taught how to mother, it is much easier to love motherhood. Today, we have to drown out the noise that sometimes does not support our choice in becoming a mother. When people spread doubt by saying things like "Can you even afford a child?" "Do you even know how to take care of a baby?" or "There goes your sleep for the next five years," these statements can rob you of your joy. It's important that your support team counteracts these statements by reassuring you that your decision was the right one and that you are going to soar as a mother. Surround yourself with those who celebrate motherhood with you. Share African-centered motherhood poems, stories, and songs, and decorate your space with beautiful art of Black mothers holding their babies. You can become a mother and still be yourself. As the famous author Toni Morrison said, "It is not true that I had to give up who I was to become a mother. It is not one or the other."[7]

It is a blessing to be a mother. This is why we celebrate it. Your personality, desires, strengths, and dislikes do not disappear because you become a mother. You will discover new perspectives and build new skills, but these only add to who you already are. I always tell people that I was already a diva before I became a mother, and I was already mothering the sick animals I found as a youth, as well as my baby nieces and cousins. Having a baby does transform you, but more in the sense that it adds to or brings out your positive qualities. For me, the feeling of being a new mother was unique each time I gave birth, and I cannot express in words the love I felt for my new baby because it was a powerful and spiritual feeling, but I am not a different person. I still enjoy the same foods, music, and dancing. I still talk fast and want to be involved with everything. That is the personality I was born with and the gifts God gave me to bring to the world, and being a mother does not dismiss that.

A lot of postpartum anxiety can come about from women wondering who they are now that they have a baby. They're stressed that they have lost themselves, and they are now "only" a mother, a shameful, lowly, and insignificant position where you have no life and your only purpose is to respond to the needs of your baby, day and night. In African American culture, it is believed that every individual is born with a spiritual purpose for being on the earth. Motherhood cannot alter this; it can only add to it. For those women who choose to birth and can birth, motherhood is an add-on to their purpose, but it does not define them.

Reconsider the notion that having a baby defines you, or that motherhood takes away your identity. You are the same amazing person you were before being pregnant, and like when you earn a degree, you only add new credentials behind your name because you always come first. Try not to measure your postpartum experience by your birth experience. Though the reproductive cycle is one, it has separate paths. Enter motherhood with joy and recognize it as an addition to your perfect self.

We must also validate that it is normal to love your baby unconditionally and intensely. These are normal, biological emotions designed to safeguard your infant until they can defend themselves. New mothers are naturally protective, so it is normal for you to want to keep your baby nearby, look at their beautiful face for hours, smell them, pick them up immediately when they cry, and offer your breast to soothe them. Most mothers naturally do not want strangers to hold their baby, nor do they want to leave their infant to return to work. New mothers are often shamed in Western culture for wanting to be stay-at-home moms or wanting to keep their new infant with them. Western culture encourages the mother to leave the baby early, whether it's for work or a date night. But science has proven that the composition of moms' brains change during pregnancy, so many are happy and content to just be with their infant, and most are not interested in a date night. A new mother would rather hold and smell her baby, like most mammals do.

If you do not feel this overwhelming love and desire to connect with your baby, that is a sign that you need more care, love, protection, and support. After the baby is born, it's important to show yourself compassion in everything that you do because you and your baby need time to adjust to each other. This can be challenging if you have other children or if your new baby cries more or has colic. Giving yourself compassion and staying patient with yourself, particularly when societal norms promote perfection, independence, and rushing, can absolutely help with your transition into motherhood. The goal is for you to slow down and savor the time with your newborn. You must stop saying, "I am a bad mother," and replace it with "I am a loving mother." This does not mean you are a perfect mother, as perfection does not exist in humans, but it does mean that you are doing the best you can. Embrace kindness, tolerance, and forgiveness toward yourself as your family and caretakers exuberate a warm, light, down-to-earth approach to help reduce your stress. Every mother has the right to expect love, peace, and happiness in her postpartum period, and you are no different.

In his book *Pyramids of Power! An Ancient African Centered Approach to Optimal Health*, Dr. John T. Chissell reiterates the spiritual belief of our ancient ancestors that God is love. Stay the course to achieve postpartum wellness by believing that you are a blessing, a sacred and special person, and surrender to the new journey. For forty-two days, go with the flow using unconditional love and trust that you are being guided and healed with pure love. Take this time to get to know your body, your emotions, and your spirit, and to love your baby. There is nothing but love in your home, so love the experience and know that love is medicine.

TIPS FOR SHOWING YOURSELF THE ULTIMATE OF LOVE

Learning to show love for yourself may be new to you, but you are deserving of reaping the benefits of this powerful healing. Here are a few steps you can take to show yourself love:

- Say daily affirmations.
- Oil your face and body with your favorite oil.
- Play your favorite songs or listen to positive podcasts.
- Laugh, watch comedy, invite your best friend over.
- Sing or hum.
- Cuddle with your partner.
- Eat warming and yummy soups.
- Flip through home-beautifying magazines.
- Revisit the Celebrate Your Beauty section in chapter 3 (pages 80–81) to remind yourself of your beauty, strength, and power.

Our postpartum rituals ignite our core instincts of being surrounded by ancient wisdom, love, and protection; the entire system is designed to provide divine healing with the sole intention of honoring the feminine and celebrating the new mother. As Toni Morrison described in a 1981 Essence interview: "Black women [need to] pay . . . attention to the ancient properties—which for me means the ability to be 'the ship' and the 'safe harbor.' Our history as Black women is the history of women who could build a house and have some children, and there was no problem. . . . What we have known is how to be complete human beings so that we did not let education keep us from our nurturing abilities. . . . [T]o lose that is to diminish ourselves unnecessarily. It is not a question, it's not a conflict. You don't have to give up anything. You choose your responsibilities."

PART THREE

Recipes and Rituals

CHAPTER 10

Recipes for Healing, Strength, and Beauty

Food is a sacred medicine. It is a blessing and gift from God. We are grateful for the elements that allowed it to grow and for the heart and hands that farmed it to be on my plate.

AFTER MUCH RESEARCH, INCLUDING READING ORAL HISTORIES OF Black postpartum rituals, studying foods of the African Diaspora, traveling in US Southern states, and sitting at the feet of Granny Midwives, I developed African American postpartum recipes for the lying-in period. My postpartum recipes include some foods that originated in Africa and historically kept Black women healthy after they birthed their babies in the United States. These recipes are the foundation that will help create wellness in the lying-in time and the first postpartum year. If you are still lactating, follow the postpartum diet for twenty-four months or longer.

These recipes combine African American and African dishes and provide hydration, protein, iron, fats, and all the other essential vitamins and minerals for good health. Plus, they are delicious! From a historical perspective, preparing food for a new mother connects us to our ancestors. Many of these recipes have been passed from generation to generation, and act as healing rituals for celebrating the new mother and baby.

THE HEALING ESSENTIALS

African American postpartum recipes include soups and stews with protein, vegetables, and fat, as well as medicinal teas and desserts laden with spices. The traditional African American postpartum diet was organic, wild, and locally sourced, but I understand if you're not able to eat this way now. Buy the freshest food possible from local farmers' markets, neighbors, or a community garden. If you cannot buy fresh, then use frozen or sodium-free canned vegetables. If you can only find salted canned food, rinse the food off before using it. Above all else, prepare these recipes with intention, prayer, and love.

Keep Potlikker on Hand

Granny Midwives always kept this traditional African American staple on hand, as it is considered a powerful postpartum food. Serve it to the mother as a warm drink, use it to cook other foods, such as rice, grits, and smashed potatoes, or add it to other soups as a base.

Be Creative

In her book *Vibration Cooking*, culinary anthropologist, griot, poet, and food writer Vertamae Smart-Grosvenor says, "Soul food is more than chitlins and greens and black-eyed peas, it's about a people who have a lot of heart and soul. . . . And when I cook, I never measure or weigh anything. I cook by vibration."[1] African American meals originated from creativity as our ancestors worked to make healthy African dishes from minimal resources during enslavement. Through ancestral memory, we acknowledged food as a blessing and used it to commemorate events, like birth, and indulge in its deliciousness. We have been given the freedom from our ancestors to mix and match, add a pinch and taste, and stir just right for the perfect postpartum healing foods. You can substitute all meats to your preference and combine meats, poultry, shellfish, and fish in one recipe. Think in color, purpose, and textures. Use the following food list to create your own unique recipes. Cook from your soul!

Many of these foods were brought from Africa to America, and we continued to use them. Try to use them in your diet to support your postpartum recuperation.

Ackee tree

Aloe—Sudan

Anise

Bananas—Wolof of Senegambia

Beans

African locust bean (Parkia biglobosa)—The seeds of this tree are fermented to produce a seasoning called dawadawa or iru, a staple in West African cooking.

Marama bean (Tylosema esculentum)—Native to Southern Africa, these protein-rich legumes are drought-resistant and offer an important food source in arid climates.

Hyacinth bean (Lablab purpureus)—Native to Africa, these beans are used both as food and fodder, and they have traditional medicinal applications in some regions.

Black-eyed peas

Boer goat

Castor bean (Ricinus communis)—Also known as castor oil, this bean is native to East Africa in Ethiopia.

Catnip—Africa

Coconut

Coffee—Ethiopia

Coriander—North Africa, mainly Morocco

Devil's claw root (Harpagophytum procumbens)—
  Namibia

Garlic—Africa

Geranium flower (Pelargonium sidoides)—South Africa

Guinea corn (Sorghum bicolor)—aka sorghum, Eastern
  Sudan

Guinea hen/fowl (Numididae)

Hibiscus (or roselle)—West Africa

Hot peppers

Kola

Lettuce (Lactuca sativa)—East African Khemit/Egyptians
  are believed to have been the first to develop this plant
  for more palatable flavors than the bitter taste of the first
  wild varieties.

Malagueta pepper (hot)—West Africa

Millet—East Africa

Myrrh (Commiphora Myrrha)—Egypt

Okra or gumbo—Okra is native to East Africa. The word
  "gumbo" is derived from a Western African word meaning "okra."

Oregano—Africa

Palm oil—West Africa

Peanuts (goobers)—West Africa

Peppermint—This plant was discovered in East Africa
  (Egypt).

Pigeon peas—Angola

Rice—The Oryza glaberrima rice species originated in West Africa.[2]

Rooibos—South Africa

Rosemary—Africa

Sesame seed (Benne)—Originates from sub-Saharan Africa

Shea butter (Butyrospermum Parkii)

Sweet basil (Ocimum basilicum)—Basil is native to tropical regions in central Africa.

Tamarind (Tamarindus indica)—Native to tropical Africa

Teff (Zuccagni)—Ethiopian

Thyme—Egypt, North Africa

Watermelon—Originated in West Africa

Yams—Native to Africa[3]

COMMON AFRICAN AMERICAN INGREDIENTS

The Granny Midwives used many foods that originated in Africa to keep mothers nourished during their postpartum period. Use what makes sense and is available to you when making your postpartum foods.

Greens: Collard, Mustard, Turnip, Kale, Poke leaves, Beet tops, Dandelion leaves, Lamb's quarters, Lettuce, Pigweed, Purslane, Rape, Rhubarb, Spinach, Watercress, Wild greens

Vegetables: Red beets, Carrots, Celery, Garlic, Golden beets, Onions, Parsnips, Radishes, White potatoes, Rutabaga, Sweet potatoes, Turnips, Parsnips, Burdock root, Okra, Corn, Cucumber, Dandelion roots, Eggplant, Green bell peppers, Hot peppers

Squashes: Butternut squash, Pumpkin squash, Yellow squash

Fruits: Apples, Bananas, Berries, Dates, Figs, Grapefruits, Grapes, Lemons, Limes, Oranges, Peaches, Plums, Prunes, Raisins, Strawberries, Tomato, Watermelon

Beans/Peas: Butter beans, Kidney beans, Lima beans, Pink beans, Snap beans, Black-eyed peas, Green peas

Nuts: Peanuts, Coconut, Pecans, Walnuts

Vinegar: White vinegar, Apple cider vinegar, Pepper vinegar

Poultry: Guinea fowl, Chicken, Turkey, Duck, Quail, Eggs

Red Meat: Beef, Deer, Goat, Lamb

Wild Game: Possum, Rabbit, Racoon, Turkey, Turtle, Rattlesnake, etc.

Shellfish: Clams, Crabs, Mussels, Oysters, Prawns, Shrimp, Lobster, Snails

Herbs and Spices: Tulsi basil, Bay leaf, Cayenne pepper, Chilis, Curry, Oregano, Salt, Thyme, Ginger, Hot pepper, Black pepper

Oils: Peanut oil, Palm oil, Coconut oil, Sesame oil, Shea butter, Olive oil, Vegetable oil

Grains: Grits, Oatmeal, Rice, Wheat, Cornmeal

Breads: Hoecakes, Hot-water cornbread, Oven cornbread, Flour biscuits, Soda crackers, Yeast bread, Hush puppies, Dumplings

Fermented Foods: Cha-cha, Buttermilk, Pickles, Pickled beets, Watermelon rind

Drinks: Dandelion-chicory-root coffee, Coffee, Green tea (sweet tea), Herbal tea, Mineral water, Spring water, Watermelon juice, Sassafras tea

Sweeteners: Cane sugar, Coconut sugar, Honey, Molasses, Sorghum syrup

Note: Besides desserts, sweetener can be added to beverages and soups to deepen or amplify flavor. If you are going to use sweetener, consider using coconut sugar for its health benefits. It contains small amounts of minerals, like iron, zinc, calcium, and potassium, along with antioxidants, such as polyphenols and flavonoids. It also has a lower glycemic index (around thirty-five to forty-five) compared to white sugar (sixty-five), meaning it may cause a slower rise in blood sugar levels. Additionally, coconut sugar contains inulin, a type of fiber that can support digestive health.[4]

SOUP IS *THE* AFRICAN AMERICAN POSTPARTUM FOOD

Known as one-pot meals, soups and stews can traced back to Africa, where it was common to cook all foods, like proteins, vegetables, and spices, together in a large pot of water. In addition to taste, these meals are full of protein, vitamins, and minerals. Adding meat and bones increases these nutritional properties. The base of most African American soups is onions, garlic, carrots, bell peppers, celery, tomatoes, bay leaves, thyme, vinegar, salt, and pepper. Soup is one of the easiest meals to make: Sauté onion and garlic in two tablespoons of oil until tender, fill the pot three quarters of the way with water, add meat (or other protein source), and bring it to a boil. Then, turn the heat down to a simmer for one hour until everything is cooked, adding diced vegetables and beans until they're soft. I usually stir in my seasoning (salt, pepper, bay leaf, thyme, curry) in the last thirty minutes. This allows the flavor to be adjusted to taste.

Though postpartum foods are meant to be soft for easy digestion, they still have enough fiber from all the vegetables to aid digestion. The meat should be so tender that it falls off the bone. When I make soup for postpartum households, I usually cook the seasoned meat until tender in the soup pot, then add my vegetables and legumes, such as black-eyed peas, tomatoes, turnips, and season with various spices. I then let the vegetables cook until they are soft, and I let it all simmer together for thirty minutes to strengthen the flavor. I then turn off the heat and let everything cool down and continue to merge flavors until it's ready to serve. Then, I serve the hot soup in a bowl or a half-full coffee mug. Because most mugs are sixteen ounces, I prefer to start new mothers off with eight ounces of soup, and because most coffee mugs maintain the heat of liquids, the soup will stay warm longer.

Black folks take a lot of pride in feeding people, and we expect to get a good response from those we feed so we know they enjoyed the food. African American postpartum foods are meant to be equal parts nutritious, healing, and delicious. Charles D. reminded me of our saying that we have to solidify this concept: "When you put your whole heart and soul into something . . . we call it putting your foot in it." So when a meal tastes good, instead of simply saying so, people will say, "You put your foot in this!" This is the ultimate compliment of a good meal!

Mama Shafia's Tips for Preparing African American Postpartum Meals

- *All food should be washed before cooking. Wash your fruits and vegetables in a bowl of lukewarm water and add a dab of liquid vegetable soap. Wash and rinse farm eggs with warm water and pat dry with a clean cloth. Always rinse off your meat, poultry, and fish.*
- *Prepare food in a clean environment with good intentions and love.*
- *Cook foods in a four-quart cast-iron pot.*
- *All meals should make at least four to six servings.*

- *You can always double a recipe and swap one protein or vegetable for another.*
- *Salt to taste.*
- *Increase seasonings to the mother's preference.*
- *All meals have a three- to four-day fridge life.*
- *The majority of meals can be frozen for three months.*
- *You can eat brown or white rice; however, brown rice has more nutrients.*

THE FIRST FORTY-TWO DAYS: RECIPES FOR THE LYING-IN PERIOD

. . . .

RICE PORRIDGE

SERVES UP TO 6
COOK TIME: 50 MINUTES

Historically, rice is a staple food in the African American community, and rice cereal is a common postpartum morning meal. Normally, it is a simple meal, but I encourage you to build it up with roasted or warmed seeds, like sesame, pecans, and walnuts; dried fruits, like prunes dates, raisins, cranberries; or fresh fruits, like peaches, sliced apples, or bananas.

INGREDIENTS

2 eggs
½ teaspoon salt
1 teaspoon nutmeg
1 teaspoon real vanilla extract
½ cup raw coconut sugar

1 cup day-old (preferable) or fresh-cooked rice
2 tablespoons butter
3 cups milk, scalded
1 cup warmed milk or coconut milk

DIRECTIONS
Preheat the oven to 350°F (175°C).

In a large bowl, lightly beat eggs, add salt, nutmeg, and vanilla extract, and stir. In a separate bowl, combine the coconut sugar and rice, and once mixed, add to the bowl of eggs.

Add butter to the scalded milk. Once the butter melts into the milk, pour into the bowl of rice and stir. Place it all into a buttered pan and bake for 45–50 minutes. After the first 15 minutes, take the pan out of the oven and stir several times, then put it back in the oven for the final 35 minutes.

When the rice cereal is firm, take it out of the oven and put in a porcelain cereal bowl (try to avoid eating out of plastic). Pour warm milk (or nut milk) over it until it becomes lightly soupy, like oatmeal.

Storage: Leftovers can be stored in the refrigerator for three days, or you can deep-freeze them for one month.

. . . .

OATMEAL PORRIDGE AND POACHED EGGS

SERVES 4–6
COOK TIME: 90 MINUTES

Oatmeal is an easy meal to make for a new mother, with a lot of different options to add in to build taste and nutrition. Porridge made from oats was a staple breakfast dish, often served with milk, raw honey, coconut sugar, or molasses. When served with poached eggs, this meal provides mamas with the fat and protein they need for optimal healing.

INGREDIENTS

¼ teaspoon salt	2 tablespoons unsalted butter
4 cups cold water	1 teaspoon cinnamon
2 cups rolled oats	2 tablespoons honey or coconut sugar
2 eggs	1 cup warm whole milk
1 tablespoon of butter	1 sliced ripe banana

DIRECTIONS

Add salt to 4 cups of simmering water and sprinkle in 2 cups of rolled oats. Cover the pot and let simmer for 30 minutes, then reduce the heat to low and simmer for 60 minutes, or until the oatmeal is thoroughly done.

While the oatmeal simmers, make the eggs. Fill a cast-iron pan with enough cold water to cover the eggs by three inches. Add 2 raw eggs, turn on the burner, and let the water simmer until the eggs become firmly cooked, for 4 to 5 minutes.

When the oatmeal is done, add it to a cereal bowl along with butter, cinnamon, and honey, stir together, then add warm milk and banana. The oatmeal should be creamy. If it's not, add a little more warm milk and stir. Serve warm with the eggs on separate plate.

Tip: You can swap bananas for raisins, dates, or prunes. You can exchange cow milk for coconut, almond, or another plant milk of your choice.

CHICKEN VEGETABLE SOUP

SERVES 4
COOK TIME: 90 MINUTES

Chicken soup has great healing power. It is considered medicinal throughout many cultures and was highly praised in ancient Egypt. Physician Moses Maimonides was known to prescribe chicken soup as a medicinal remedy for colds and asthma.[5] I love to make a double batch of this so families can freeze half and eat it later.

INGREDIENTS

1 whole chicken, head and feet removed
½ teaspoon salt
½ teaspoon black pepper to taste
1 teaspoon garlic powder
4 tablespoons peanut oil (or vegetable oil of your choice)
1 medium onion, diced
4 garlic cloves, minced
5 celery stalks, diced

1 large green bell pepper, diced
8 cups water
5 carrots, diced
1 small bag of frozen peas
2 bay leaves, halved
3 thyme twigs with leaves
1 teaspoon cayenne pepper to taste
1 teaspoon white vinegar
1 teaspoon sugar or honey

DIRECTIONS

Season the outside and inside of the chicken with salt, black pepper, and garlic powder, then let sit for 30 minutes.

Pour peanut oil in a four-quart cast-iron stock pot, heat on medium-high, then add onion, garlic, celery, and green bell pepper. Sauté until soft (3–5 minutes). Remove the sauteed vegetables and set aside. Put chicken in the pot and brown for 5–7 minutes on each side, adding more oil if needed to prevent burning.

Once the chicken is browned, add water, carrots, sauteed vegetables, frozen peas, and bay leaves to the pot. Simmer for 30 minutes.

Once the chicken is cooked, turn off the heat. Safely remove the chicken from the pot and place it into a bowl of ice-cold water. Once the chicken is cooled down, take it out of the cold water and let it sit on a cutting board for 10 minutes. Remove and discard the outer skin, cut the chicken into small pieces, then add the cut chicken and bones back to the pot of water. Bring to a low simmer for 30 more minutes.

Add thyme, cayenne pepper, vinegar, and sugar, and let simmer for 20 minutes. Turn off heat, cover pot, and let soup sit for 10 minutes, then serve.

Storage: Leftovers can be stored in the refrigerator for three days, or you can deep-freeze them for one month.

PEANUT BUTTER SOUP (GROUNDNUT SOUP)

SERVES 4
COOK TIME: 60 MINUTES

Peanut butter soup is an old-timey African American recipe with roots in Africa. Peanuts, also known as goobers, contain 3.8 grams of protein per eight ounces and 2.7 grams of iron per serving. Overall, they have thirty essential vitamins and minerals, and are high in antioxidants and fiber. Because of all these nutrients, this soup is great for new mamas. Of course, make sure no one in the postpartum household has a peanut allergy before making and serving this recipe.

INGREDIENTS

1 chicken or 7 chicken parts (legs, thighs, and half wings)
1 teaspoon salt
2 teaspoons cayenne pepper
1 tablespoon curry powder
1 teaspoon ginger powder
¼ teaspoon nutmeg
1 medium onion, diced

2 garlic cloves, minced
2 bell peppers (any color), diced
1 celery stalk, chopped
Peanut oil
8 cups water
1 cup smooth, unsalted peanut butter
2 carrots, diced
½ (6-ounce) can tomato paste

DIRECTIONS

Cut the chicken into 7 pieces. Season with salt, pepper, curry, ginger, and nutmeg, then let sit.

Sauté onions, garlic, bell pepper, and celery in peanut oil for 3–5 minutes. Remove sauteed vegetables and set aside. Put the chicken pieces and brown in the same pot for 5–8 minutes.

Once the chicken is browned, add 8 cups of water to the pot and bring it to a simmer for 20 minutes.

Remove 2 cups of pot likker and mix well with peanut butter. Add peanut butter mix back to the pot, along with the sauteed vegetables, carrots, and tomato paste; stir the pot three times; and bring to a low simmer for another 30 minutes. When the soup looks smooth and you see the peanut oil rise to the top, it's done. Turn off the pot and cover. Let it sit for 10 minutes to allow the flavor to set in. You can serve it alone or over a small bowl of rice or grits.

Storage: Leftovers can be stored in the refrigerator for three days, or you can deep-freeze them for one month.

COCONUT SHRIMP SOUP

SERVES 4
COOK TIME: 30 MINUTES

Shellfish has a strong history in the Black community, resulting from the rich history of a fishing people along the shores of Africa who were brought to the Atlantic shores of the United States. Shrimp with coconut milk is a nutritious and filling soup. You can substitute fish pieces for the shrimp.

INGREDIENTS

2 cups deveined jumbo shrimp

2 teaspoons cayenne pepper

1 teaspoon salt

3 tablespoons coconut oil

1 bunch green scallions, chopped

2 celery stalks, diced

¼ cup white onions, diced

5 cups cold water

1 cup green peas

2 fresh thyme sprigs, or 1 teaspoon dried thyme

1 teaspoon chives, diced

1 bay leaf

1 cup coconut milk

1 teaspoon oyster sauce

2 teaspoons lime juice, or half a lime

DIRECTIONS

Season jumbo shrimp with cayenne pepper and salt. Let marinate while you chop and dice the scallions, celery, and onions. Melt the coconut oil over low heat in a pot, then add the vegetables, and sauté until soft (for about 5 minutes).

Remove the sauteed vegetables with a slotted spoon, add the shrimp to the pot, and sauté until cooked (for 4 to 5 minutes), then remove and add to the plate of sauteed vegetables.

Pour 5 cups of cold water in the pot, then add the sauteed vegetables back into the pot. Add the peas, thyme, chives, and bay leaf, then simmer on low for 15 minutes.

Add the coconut milk and oyster sauce to the pot and simmer for another 10 minutes. Turn off the pot and add shrimp and remove the bay leaf and thyme sprigs. Add 2 teaspoons of lime juice and stir thoroughly. Cover pot, let sit for 5 minutes, then serve.

Storage: Leftovers can be stored in the refrigerator for three days, or you can deep-freeze them for one month.

SPINACH GARLIC STEW WITH CHICKEN

SERVES 6
COOK TIME: 60 MINUTES

There is a lot of garlic in this stew—and for good reason. Garlic has many healing properties, including aiding in digestion and alleviating common cold symptoms.[6] Combined with other healing spices and chicken protein, this is a warming and nourishing stew.

INGREDIENTS

½ chicken, cut into four or five pieces

1 teaspoon cumin

2 tablespoons curry powder

¼ teaspoon ginger powder

¼ cup palm oil

1 medium white onion, diced

½ jalapeno pepper, chopped

1 garlic bulb, peeled and minced

8 cups water

½ (15-ounce) can whole tomatoes

4 cups spinach, without stems, chopped

1 teaspoon salt

2 teaspoons cayenne pepper

¼ teaspoon fresh chives

DIRECTIONS

Season chicken with the cumin, curry, and ginger.

Melt palm oil over medium heat in a four-quart pot, then sauté white onion, jalapeno, and garlic until tender (for about 5 minutes).

Add 8 cups of water and the seasoned chicken, and bring to a simmer. Add the tomatoes and let simmer for 30 minutes.

Turn heat down to low. Add spinach to the pot and let it cook down, then add salt, cayenne, and chives. Simmer for another 30 minutes, then turn off the heat and let sit for 10 minutes to allow the flavor to set in. Serve by itself in a soup bowl or over a cup of cooked rice.

Storage: This meal can be refrigerated for three days and will keep in the freezer for two weeks.

CURRIED CHICKEN, MIXED GREENS, AND COCONUT SOUP

SERVES 4
COOK TIME: 90 MINUTES

This is one of my favorite soups to jump-start the postpartum healing process. The coconut milk provides energy, hydration, and essential nutrients that support performance and recovery for uterine repair. The leafy green vegetables provide iron, vitamin K, vitamin C, folate, and cal-cium, which support bone health, immunity, and overall wellness. The collards can be replaced with mustard greens or kale.

INGREDIENTS

6 pieces of chicken (any parts)
½ teaspoon salt
2 teaspoons cayenne pepper
1 teaspoon cumin
½ cup onion, diced
3 tablespoons coconut oil
2 cups collard greens, finely chopped
2 cups turnip greens, finely chopped
7 cups water

4 tablespoons curry powder
1 teaspoon ginger powder
3 garlic cloves, minced
3 medium red tomatoes, chopped
1 (15-ounce) can coconut milk
2 teaspoons hickory liquid smoke
2 tablespoons white vinegar
½ teaspoon honey
1 teaspoon thyme

DIRECTIONS

Season the chicken with salt, cayenne pepper, and cumin, then let sit.

Sauté the onions in coconut oil for 6 to 10 minutes on low heat in a four-quart pot. Do not let them burn. Once tender, remove the onions from the pot and set aside.

Add the seasoned chicken to the pot and brown on all sides. Once browned, remove the chicken from the pot and set aside with the onions.

Put both the greens in the pot and sauté until wilted.

Add 7 cups of water to the pot and simmer for 10 minutes. Add the onions and chicken back to the pot, stir everything together, and let simmer for 30 minutes. Add the curry, ginger, cloves, and tomatoes, stir, then add coconut milk, hickory liquid smoke, vinegar, honey, and thyme, and let simmer for an additional 30 minutes. Turn off the heat, let sit for 10 minutes, then serve in a soup bowl.

Storage: This meal can be refrigerated for three days and will keep in the freezer for two weeks.

TURKEY NECK AND LIMA BEAN SOUP

SERVES 4–6
COOK TIME: 60 MINUTES

Neck bones are a traditional food, stemming from a time when using all of the animal was a way of life. Turkey necks are very nutritious as they are a good source of protein and collagen, along with other nutrients. Combined with lima beans and spices, this is another warming and nourishing meal.

INGREDIENTS

3 tablespoons flour

1 teaspoon salt

1 teaspoon black pepper

5 turkey necks

2 tablespoons unsalted butter

2–3 garlic cloves, minced

1 onion, chopped

5 celery stalks, chopped

8 cups water

1 cup frozen lima beans

1 vine ripe tomato, chopped

1 bay leaf, halved

1 teaspoon thyme

½ teaspoon cumin powder

2 teaspoons hickory liquid smoke

2 teaspoons white vinegar

1 teaspoon honey

Rice

Hot sauce to taste

DIRECTIONS

Season flour with salt and pepper, then roll the turkey necks in it. Melt butter in a pot and brown the turkey necks on all sides, with the garlic, onion, and celery.

Add water to the pot and bring to a boil for 10 minutes, then add the lima beans and tomato and simmer for another 40 minutes. During this time, add the bay leaf, thyme, cumin, cloves, hickory liquid smoke, vinegar, and honey. When the lima beans become soft, turn off the pot, remove the bay leaf, cover, then let sit for 10 minutes to allow flavors to set in. Add salt and pepper to taste and serve with rice and hot sauce.

Storage: This meal can be refrigerated for three days and will keep in the freezer for two months.

. . . .

VEGGIE BONE SOUP

SERVES 4–6

COOK TIME: 2 HOURS

This recipe calls for many beef bones, but that is the way it's been made from before the time of the Granny Midwives. This bone soup is nutritious for a new mother. It's easy to make too, so you can always keep it on hand for sipping or to use as a nutrient-rich base for other soups and stews.

INGREDIENTS

10 cups water

3 beef bones with meat on them (use the bones you prefer)

1 teaspoon salt

2 bay leaves, halved

1 teaspoon thyme

1 bell pepper, seeded and chopped

1 small yellow onion, diced

3 celery stalks with leaves, roughly chopped

½ teaspoon cumin
2 teaspoons cayenne pepper
1 medium yellow turnip, chopped
1 carrot, chopped
½ cup black-eyed peas

1 sweet potato, chopped
2 green scallions, chopped
2 teaspoons white vinegar
1 tablespoon unsalted butter

DIRECTIONS

Place water, beef bones, salt, bay leaves, and a sprig of fresh thyme in the pot, then simmer for 1 hour.

Lower the heat, add the remaining ingredients except for the butter, then let simmer for another hour. Remove bay leaves and thyme sprig.

Turn off the heat and stir the butter into the soup. Cover and let sit for 10 minutes. Serve alone or with rice.

Storage: This meal can be refrigerated for three days and will keep in the freezer for two months.

· ·

BLACK-EYED PEA, SPINACH, AND FISH SOUP

SERVES 4–6
COOK TIME: 3 HOURS

Cooking the whole fish, with the head, is still the norm for many African American families, and is traditional in many cultures. If you don't want to cook a whole fish, you can use chunks. Catfish or bass work best here, but use whatever you like.

INGREDIENTS

3 tablespoons unsalted butter
1 teaspoon salt
1 teaspoon black pepper
1 teaspoon ground thyme
3 teaspoons garlic powder
2 whole fish, with head intact
½ cup white flour
3 tablespoons peanut oil
3 garlic cloves, minced
1 medium yellow onion, diced
1 green bell pepper, seeded and chopped

1 celery stalk with leaves, chopped
10 cups water
2 bay leaves, halved
1 cup cooked black-eyed peas
1 cup okra, chopped
2 cups spinach, roughly chopped
3 large tomatoes, chopped
1 teaspoon cayenne pepper
1 thyme sprig
1 teaspoon ground ginger
1 teaspoon fresh lemon juice

DIRECTIONS

Preheat oven to 350°F (175°C).

Mix butter with salt, pepper, ground thyme, and garlic powder. Rub seasoned butter on the fish, then roll the buttered fish in white flour and bake for 20–25 minutes.

Heat peanut oil in a pot over medium heat and sauté the minced garlic, onions, green bell pepper, and celery for 5 to 7 minutes.

Add 10 cups of water to pot and simmer for 1 hour with bay leaves, sprig of thyme, black-eyed peas, okra, spinach, tomatoes, cayenne pepper, ginger, and lemon juice.

Turn off the heat, add the baked fish, cover, and let sit for 10 minutes before serving.

Storage: This meal can be refrigerated for three days and will keep in the freezer for two weeks.

WEST AFRICAN PALM OIL SOUP WITH FISH

SERVES 4–6
COOK TIME: 70 MINUTES

Palm oil is a necessary food for the postpartum period. Palm oil is rich in antioxidants and carotenoids, the base of vitamins A and E. This soup is a variation of the one I have been eating for years. It is brimming with nutrients and flavor. If you do not want to cook whole fish, you can use filets. I like to use bass for this recipe, but you can use your favorite fish.

INGREDIENTS:

1 teaspoon salt
2 whole fish
½ cup palm oil
1 medium yellow onion, chopped
3 garlic cloves, mashed
1 (15-ounce) can stewed whole tomatoes
8 cups water
2 celery ribs, chopped
1 cup chopped fresh okra

1 medium turnip, peeled and halved
1 teaspoon ginger powder, or 2 teaspoons of fresh grated ginger
2 teaspoons cayenne pepper
3 tablespoons curry powder
2 cups leafy greens (mustard, collards, turnip, pumpkin leaves, or kale will work)
Rice for serving

DIRECTIONS

Wash and salt the fish and set aside.

Heat palm oil in a pot over medium heat, add onion and garlic, and sauté for 10 minutes (do not let oil smoke).

Add the stewed tomatoes, let cook for 10 minutes, then add water, celery, okra, and turnip and bring to a low boil for 30 minutes, until vegetables are soft.

Turn the heat down to a simmer, then add ginger powder, cayenne pepper, curry powder, and the greens. Cut fish in half, add to the soup, and let simmer for 10 minutes. Serve with rice.

Storage: This meal can be refrigerated for three days and will keep in the freezer for two weeks.

· ·

OXTAIL RED BEAN SOUP

SERVES 4–6
COOK TIME: 90 MINUTES

Oxtails are considered to be offal and are also high in protein, iron, fat, minerals, and vitamins. Along with the beans, this thick soup offers double the protein—perfect to help new mamas get their strength back. You can substitute turkey necks, goat, or lamb bones as well.

INGREDIENTS

2 cups oxtails
¼ teaspoon celery salt
1 teaspoon onion powder
¼ teaspoon ginger powder
3 teaspoons hickory liquid smoke
2 teaspoons granulated garlic
1 teaspoon ground black pepper
2 tablespoons peanut oil
1 cup diced onion
3 fresh garlic cloves, smashed
1 celery stalk with leaves, chopped
1 green bell pepper, seeded and chopped
1 cup finely chopped collard greens
10 cups water

1 (15-ounce) can red kidney beans, drained and rinsed, or 2 cups freshly cooked
1 cup fresh or frozen organic corn kernels
1 carrot, chopped
1 (15-ounce) can tomato sauce
½ teaspoon thyme
1 bay leaf
¼ teaspoon cayenne pepper
2 teaspoons paprika
½ teaspoon chili powder
1 scotch bonnet pepper, seeded and minced
¼ teaspoon salt

DIRECTIONS

Season oxtails with celery salt, onion powder, ginger powder, 1 teaspoon of liquid smoke, granulated garlic, and black pepper, and set aside for 15 minutes.

Warm peanut oil in large stock pot over low heat and sauté the onions, garlic, celery, bell pepper, and collard greens for 7 to 10 minutes, stirring frequently so they don't burn. Remove from pot and set aside.

Put the seasoned oxtails in the same pot, turn the heat up to medium, and brown on all sides for 7 to 10 minutes.

Once browned, add water, the sauteed vegetables, red kidney beans, corn, carrot, and tomato sauce, and simmer for 30 minutes.

Add the thyme, bay leaf, cayenne pepper, paprika, chili powder, scotch bonnet pepper, and remaining liquid smoke, then turn the heat down and simmer for another 40 minutes, until the vegetables are soft.

Remove a half cup of beans and stock and smash the beans with a potato masher. Add the bean and broth mixture back to the pot and stir. Remove the bay leaf, turn off the heat, and let sit for 10 minutes to allow the flavor to set in. Serve hot alone or with rice.

Storage: This meal can be refrigerated for three days and will keep in the freezer for two weeks.

MORE POSTPARTUM MEALS FOR THE FIRST YEAR

The "delayed postpartum period" is from six weeks to twelve months. Postpartum nutrition is still needed during this time because muscle tone and connective tissues are still returning to their nonpregnant state, and iron stores are still being built, up to twenty-four months after birth, or until breastfeeding ends. I tell my mothers and their families to make batches of these meals to keep on hand for easy and warming nourishment.

LIVER AND FIG STEW

SERVES 4–6
COOK TIME: 60 MINUTES

Chicken livers are a traditional food that elders gave postpartum mothers to help them regain their strength. Rich in iron, this stew is especially good for treating anemia. The figs add some sweetness, along with iron, fiber, potassium, and other vitamins.

INGREDIENTS

1 cup flour
3 dashes of salt
Black pepper to taste
½ teaspoon cumin

½ teaspoon nutmeg
1 teaspoon garlic powder
¼ teaspoon powdered ginger
½ teaspoon thyme

5 chicken livers	1 tablespoon unsalted butter
3 tablespoons olive oil	5 cups water
1 medium onion, sliced into circles	2 teaspoons white vinegar
4 figs, halved	1 cup brown rice, washed

DIRECTIONS

Season flour by placing it in a brown paper bag along with salt, pepper, cumin, nutmeg, garlic powder, ginger, and thyme. Shake to combine. Season the chicken livers by adding them to the bag and shaking until they are fully coated.

Heat olive oil in a pot over medium-high heat and sauté onion and figs for 6 to 7 minutes. Drain onions and figs on a paper towel and set aside.

Put butter in the pot. When melted, brown the chicken livers to semi-cooked. Remove from the pan and let rest.

Put 2 tablespoons of the seasoned flour in the pot and brown. Slowly add one cup of water and stir constantly with a fork to prevent lumps and create a smooth gravy. Add 2 more cups of water to the gravy and let simmer for 30 minutes.

Once the gravy looks smooth, add the onions, figs, and vinegar and simmer for 20 minutes.

Turn off the heat, add the liver, cover, and let sit for 10 minutes. It should be a wet stew gravy at this point.

Make the rice. Bring 2 cups of water to a simmer in a separate pot and add brown rice. Let simmer until the water has evaporated, stir rice once, then remove from heat, cover, and let steam until the rice is soft.

Serve the stew over a bowl of rice.

Storage: This meal can be refrigerated for seven days. It will not freeze well.

. . . .

SUCCOTASH STEW

SERVES 4–5
COOK TIME: 60 MINUTES

A traditional meal with Native American origins, succotash is traditionally made with corn and lima beans. I like to add shrimp for extra taste and nutrients.

INGREDIENTS

| 2 tablespoons peanut oil | ½ cup finely diced white onion |

3 garlic cloves, minced

¼ cup seeded and diced green bell pepper

¼ jalapeno pepper, seeded and diced

5 cups water

½ teaspoon celery salt

½ teaspoon dried thyme

½ cup frozen or fresh lima beans

2 tomatoes, sliced

1 cup okra, sliced into rounds

1 teaspoon black pepper

1 cup shelled shrimp, deveined

Juice of ¼ large lemon, or 1–1 ½ teaspoons lemon juice

3 teaspoons Worcestershire sauce

2 teaspoons honey

8 shakes of Louisiana hot sauce

Rice for serving

DIRECTIONS

Heat peanut oil on medium heat, then sauté onion, garlic, bell pepper, and jalapeno for 5 to 7 minutes on low heat, until soft and barely browned.

Add water, celery salt, thyme, lima beans, and tomatoes, and bring to a boil. Once it's boiling, turn heat to medium and let simmer for 20 minutes.

Add okra, black pepper, and deveined shrimp, then turn heat down and let simmer for 30 minutes.

Turn off heat and add lemon juice, Worcestershire sauce, and honey, and stir to combine fully.

Let set for 10 minutes, then shake in hot sauce. Serve with brown or white enriched rice.

Storage: This meal can be refrigerated for three days and will keep in the freezer for two months.

. . . .

BROWNED GOAT STEW

SERVES 6

COOK TIME: 2 HOURS

Goat, considered a red meat, is used in a lot of traditional African recipes due to its abundance. I prefer goat over lamb because it is a leaner meat. Goat is also higher in protein and iron. The secret to taming goat's gamey taste is to preseason it and cook it low and slow. If you don't like goat or it isn't available, you can use beef, lamb, or chicken instead.

INGREDIENTS

3 pounds goat (bone-in)

2 teaspoons onion powder

2 teaspoons cumin

2 teaspoons dried thyme

½ teaspoon paprika

1 teaspoon black pepper

½ teaspoon salt

½ teaspoon cayenne pepper

4 tablespoons peanut oil

¼ cup chopped yellow onion

5 garlic cloves, minced
3 celery stalks, chopped
4 tablespoons white flour
6 cups water

5 ripe tomatoes
2 bay leaves, halved
1 cup unpeeled cubed purple eggplant
2 teaspoons cane sugar

DIRECTIONS

Preseason goat pieces. Place goat in a glass bowl and season with onion powder, cumin, thyme, paprika, black pepper, salt, and cayenne pepper. Massage spices into goat for 3 minutes. Cover the bowl and let sit for 30 minutes. *Tip: For faster cooking, preseason the meat the night before and let it sit in the fridge until you're ready to cook.*

Heat peanut oil in a cast-iron pot on medium heat, and sauté onion, garlic, and celery for 5 to 7 minutes, or until soft. Remove sauteed vegetables from pot and place in a glass bowl.

Sprinkle flour on the marinated goat and toss it so it's fully coated. Turn heat to medium-high, then once the seasoned peanut oil is lightly hot, add the goat and brown on all sides. Stir occasionally with a wooden spoon to prevent the goat from burning. If needed, you can add a little more peanut oil.

Once the goat is browned, add cold water to the pot. Bring water to a boil for 30 minutes, then reduce the heat to low and simmer for 1 hour, or until goat becomes very tender. Once tender, add the tomatoes, bay leaves, and eggplant. Bring to a boil for 5 minutes, then lower the heat, add sugar, and simmer for 30 minutes. Turn off the heat, cover the pot, and let sit for 10 minutes. Serve on its own or with rice.

Storage: This meal can be refrigerated for three days and will keep in the freezer for three months.

BEEF STEW

SERVES 6
COOK TIME: 2 HOURS
This hearty stew has lots of protein, iron, calcium, fiber, and other minerals. It's filling, warming, nourishing, and is also good for hydration—perfect to help you regain your strength.

INGREDIENTS

½ pound cubed beef
Salt
2 teaspoons onion powder
1 teaspoon chili powder
1 tablespoon curry powder
1 teaspoon ground black pepper

½ teaspoon cayenne pepper
4 tablespoons olive oil
½ cup chopped onion
5 garlic cloves, minced
½ cup chopped celery with leaves
1 jalapeno, seeded and diced

8 cups water
1 bay leaf
3 medium-sized carrots, sliced in
medium-sized circles
2 red bell peppers, seeded and sliced

1 sweet potato, cubed
1 cup cooked black-eyed peas
2 teaspoons hickory liquid smoke
1 teaspoon raw sugar

DIRECTIONS

In a large glass bowl, season beef with salt, onion powder, chili powder, curry powder, black pepper, and cayenne and massage into the meat for 3 minutes. Set aside and marinate for 1 hour.

In a medium pot over medium-high heat, sauté the marinated beef in olive oil until brown on all sides. Remove the meat with a slotted spoon.

Place onion, garlic, celery, and jalapeno pepper in the pot and sauté.

Once the vegetables are soft, add 8 cups of cold water to the pot, add the beef back in, add the bay leaf, carrots, bell pepper, sweet potato, black-eyed peas, liquid smoke, and sugar, and let simmer for 2 hours.

Turn off the heat and let sit for 10 minutes. Serve in a ceramic bowl or large cup plain or with a bit of rice.

Storage: This meal can be refrigerated for three days and will keep in the freezer for two months.

. . . .

HOPPIN' JOHN SHRIMP STEW

SERVES 4–6
COOK TIME: 2 HOURS

This popular dish is served for good luck on New Year's Day, but every day is a blessing for new mothers, so we offer Hoppin' John Shrimp Stew any day of the year.[7]

INGREDIENTS

3 tablespoons coconut oil
1 medium white onion, chopped
3 garlic cloves, minced
2 celery stalks, finely diced
5 cups water
1 cup turnip or mustard greens, finely
chopped
1 cup frozen black-eyed peas
1 large tomato, chopped

2 teaspoons hickory liquid smoke
1 teaspoon Worcestershire sauce
1 teaspoon cayenne pepper
½ teaspoon cumin
1 teaspoon paprika
1 teaspoon ground black pepper
½ teaspoon salt
2 teaspoons cane sugar
1 bay leaf, halved

1 cup shelled shrimp (can be replaced with fish or meat)

½ cup coconut oil

2 teaspoons cayenne pepper

DIRECTIONS

Over medium-high heat, melt coconut oil in a large pot. Add onions, garlic, and celery, and sauté until soft (for about 5 minutes).

Add water and bring to a simmer. Add chopped greens and continue simmering for 60 minutes.

Add black-eyed peas, tomato, liquid smoke, Worcestershire sauce, cayenne pepper, cumin, paprika, black pepper, salt, sugar, and bay leaf, and let cook for another hour.

Add shrimp and simmer for 15 minutes, then turn off heat. Cover the pot, let sit for 10 minutes, then serve. (Rice is optional.)

Storage: This meal can be refrigerated for three days or placed in the freezer for three months.

. . . .

PEPPER AND HOMINY GRIT STEW

SERVES 4–6
COOK TIME: 90 MINUTES

Hominy grits are made from corn and were a major staple for new mothers in the nineteenth and twentieth centuries. I love to serve mamas a bowl of hominy grit stew garnished with hot sauce, chives, and a parsley sprig.

INGREDIENTS

4 cups water

1 teaspoon salt

1 cup stoneground course yellow cornmeal/grits

1 stick unsalted butter

½ cup grated sharp cheddar cheese

1½ teaspoons fresh ground black peppercorns

2 beef or chicken sausages, halved vertically

½ onion, chopped

½ green bell pepper, seeded and chopped

3 garlic cloves, minced

¼ cup dried chives

1 sprig fresh parsley

¼ cup cooked black-eyed peas

1 tablespoon red hot sauce

DIRECTIONS

For the grits: Bring water and salt to a boil in a four-quart pot. Lower the heat and stir in grits. Stir constantly to prevent lumps and cook for 45 to 60 minutes. Once grits look smooth, stir in ¾ of the stick of butter, cheese, and pepper, cover, and let simmer for another 5 to 10 minutes.

In a cast-iron skillet over medium-high heat, melt the remaining butter and brown the sausages on both sides (for about 5 minutes on each side) and cook thoroughly for another 3 minutes. Once cooked, remove the sausages from the skillet and sauté the onions, green bell pepper, garlic, chives, parsley, and black-eyed peas until softened (for about 7 to 10 minutes). Add the sausages back to the skillet, stir, and heat up. Serve grits in a bowl with hot sauce, a ½ cup of vegetables and two sausage halves on top. Garnish with fresh chives and serve.

Storage: This meal can be refrigerated for three to five days and frozen for up to three months.

GREEN BEAN AND BROWN CHICKEN STEW

SERVES 4–6
COOK TIME: 60 MINUTES

Growing up, my grandmother referred to green beans as "snapped beans" because of the distinct snap sound they made when we broke them in half. They are a great source of folate and fiber for the postpartum mother.

INGREDIENTS

5 chicken parts
½ cup flour, seasoned with salt and pepper
¼ cup olive oil
6 cups water
2 cups green beans, snapped in half
1 bay leaf, halved
2 celery stalks, diced small
2 onions, chopped

2 garlic cloves, minced
2 tomatoes, cubed
1 cup tomato sauce
1 jalapeno, seeded and chopped
½ teaspoon black pepper
½ (15-ounce) can coconut cream
2 teaspoons vinegar
1 teaspoon salt

DIRECTIONS

Lightly coat chicken in seasoned flour. Heat oil in cast-iron skillet, add chicken, and brown on all sides (for about 5 minutes on each side). Pour water in a four-quart pot, then add green beans, bay leaf, celery, onions, and garlic, and bring to a boil for 10 minutes. Skim off any foam, then lower the heat and add the tomatoes, tomato sauce, jalapeno, and black pepper. Simmer until the beans are tender and the chicken is done (for about 40 minutes).

Shake the can of coconut cream, then add half the can and the vinegar to the pot. Let simmer for another 10 minutes.

Turn off the heat, remove the bay leaf, add salt to taste, and serve hot in a soup bowl.

Storage: This meal can be refrigerated for three days and will keep in the freezer for three months.

LAMB, KALE, POTATO STEW

SERVES 4–6
COOK TIME: 2 HOURS

Lamb is another meat that some people may not like, though I say that they probably just haven't had the right recipe. Lamb is incredibly nutritious and rich in iron, zinc, and vitamin B-12. It does have a lot of fat that needs to be poured off before combining with other ingredients. Lamb works well with greens, scallions, and sweet potato in this stew.

INGREDIENTS

2 cups lamb meat with bone
Salt to taste
2 teaspoons ginger powder
1 teaspoon black pepper
3 tablespoons olive oil
1 small white onion, diced
1 red bell pepper, seeded and chopped
5 garlic cloves, minced
4 large mushrooms (any available), diced

2 cups kale, finely chopped (can be replaced with collard, mustard, or turnip greens)
5 cups water
2 tomatoes, chopped
2 tablespoons curry powder
½ teaspoon cumin
1 teaspoon cayenne pepper
2 medium sweet potatoes, cut in fourths

DIRECTIONS

In a shallow dish, marinate lamb pieces with salt, ginger, and dashes of black pepper for 30 minutes, then bake in oven until tender and cooked. Put olive oil in a large pot, and sauté the onion, bell pepper, garlic, and mushrooms over low heat.

Add the kale and stir for 5 minutes.

Add water to the pot and let simmer on low heat. Next, remove lamb from oven and place on paper towels to absorb the excess fat. Then, add lamb pieces to the pot and continue to simmer. Add the tomatoes, curry powder, cumin, and cayenne pepper, and let simmer for 1 hour. Then, add the sweet potatoes and let cook for 15 minutes. When potatoes are soft, usually when you can easily pierce them with a fork, turn off the heat, cover the pot, and let sit for 10 minutes to allow the flavors to set in.

Serve hot.

Storage: This meal can be refrigerated for three to seven days and will keep in the freezer for three months.

BEEF AND TURNIP STEW

SERVES 4–6
COOK TIME: 80–90 MINUTES

Turnip greens are a bit more tender than collard greens, so you can cook them in less time. Besides being tender, they offer important vitamins and minerals, such as calcium and vitamin K, which can help new mamas in their postpartum recuperation.[8]

INGREDIENTS

5 tablespoons peanut oil
2 cups stewed beef cubes
1 medium yellow onion, diced
1 garlic clove, diced
5 cups water
2 cups turnip greens
1 turnip, cut in fourths
2 carrots, peeled and chopped

Salt
Black pepper
2 teaspoons white vinegar
1 teaspoon honey
1 teaspoon thyme
1 tablespoon hickory liquid smoke
Rice for serving

DIRECTIONS

In a large pot, heat peanut oil on medium-high heat, then sauté the seasoned beef cubes with onion and garlic until the aromatics become clear (for about 5 minutes).

Add water, turnip greens, turnip, and carrots, and let simmer for about 50 minutes.

When it is nearly done, add salt, black pepper, white vinegar, honey, thyme, and liquid smoke. Stir and let cook for 20 minutes.

Remove from heat, cover, and let sit for 10 minutes, then serve with rice.

Storage: This meal can be refrigerated for three to seven days and will keep in the freezer for three months.

PALM OIL SOUP

SERVES 6
COOK TIME: 90 MINUTES

Palm oil comes from West Africa, and it is a nutrient-rich powerhouse full of vitamins and minerals. I love palm oil soup and make it for my family at least three times per month. You can purchase palm oil at African stores or some organic food stores. It's worth consuming palm oil soup in the postpartum stage for the health benefits.

INGREDIENTS

6 cubes of goat with the bone intact
1 teaspoon salt
2 teaspoons ground black pepper
1 medium yellow onion, diced
5 garlic cloves, diced
½ cup palm oil
2 tablespoons palm oil
8 cups water
1 bay leaf, halved

1 teaspoon dried thyme
½ teaspoon ginger powder
3 tablespoons curry powder
2 tablespoons chopped chives
2 cups precooked black-eyed peas
1 green bell pepper, sliced into small pieces
1 (15-ounce) can whole tomatoes
2 teaspoons cayenne pepper

DIRECTIONS

Cover goat with salt and black pepper and let sit as you dice the onion and garlic.

Next, melt the palm oil in a four-quart pot over medium heat. Sauté the onion and garlic until they become clear, then add the water followed by the seasoned goat. Bring to a low boil for 30 minutes. After 30 minutes, add the bay leaf, thyme, ginger, curry, chives, black-eyed peas, and green bell pepper, and let cook for another 15 minutes. Add the tomatoes and cayenne pepper, and cook for an additional 30 minutes. Turn off the heat, cover, and let sit for 10 minutes. Serve in a bowl with rice or alone.

Storage: This meal can be refrigerated for three days and will keep in the freezer for two months.

. . . .

SWEET POTATO, GINGER, CHICKEN SOUP

SERVES 4–6
COOK TIME: 90 MINUTES

Sweet potatoes are rich in vitamin A, potassium, and other nutrients and provide a good amount of energy for postpartum mothers.[9]

INGREDIENTS

4 chicken legs
½ teaspoon salt
½ teaspoon black pepper
3 tablespoons butter
1 medium white onion, chopped
2 garlic cloves, minced
1 celery stalk, chopped
5 cups chicken stock, fresh or canned

1 cup turnip greens, roughly chopped
2 cups peeled and cubed sweet potatoes
¼ teaspoon ground cinnamon
2 tablespoons minced fresh ginger
1 tablespoon honey
1 teaspoon non-GMO soy sauce
1 teaspoon white vinegar
Rice for serving

DIRECTIONS

Season chicken legs with salt and pepper. Melt butter in a large pot on medium heat, then brown the chicken on all sides. Remove from the pot and set aside.

Put the onion, garlic, and celery in the pot and sauté until soft (for 5 to 7 minutes).

Add the chicken stock and bring to a simmer. Add the turnip greens and continue simmering for 1 hour.

Add the sweet potatoes and cook until fork-tender (for about 20 minutes).

Add cinnamon, ginger, honey, soy sauce, and vinegar. Stir, turn off the heat, and cover. Let sit for 10 minutes. Serve with rice.

Storage: This meal can be refrigerated for three days and will keep in the freezer for three months.

. . . .

SEAFOOD GUMBO

SERVES 6
COOK TIME: 2 HOURS

This gumbo is warming, satisfying, and great for increasing strength. Do not eat if you are allergic to shellfish!

INGREDIENTS

½ pound each of shrimp, mussels, clams, and/or crab legs
8 cups water
2 bay leaves, halved
¼ teaspoon dried thyme
½ teaspoon dried basil
½ teaspoon dried marjoram
1 teaspoon salt
Black pepper to taste
½ pound beef sausage, sliced
½ stick unsalted butter
2 celery stalks with leaves, chopped
1 medium yellow onion, diced
2 garlic cloves, minced

2 cups carrots, cut into 1-inch pieces
1 large, firm green bell pepper, seeded and chopped into 1-inch pieces
½ cup all-purpose organic white flour
1 (15-ounce) can whole tomatoes
1 (15-ounce) can black-eyed peas, or 1 cup freshly cooked
Hot peppers to taste (you can use a jalapeno, seeded and diced, or 1 teaspoon cayenne powder)
3 parsley stalks, chopped
1 teaspoon Worcestershire sauce
1 teaspoon oyster sauce

DIRECTIONS

Wash seafood, remove shells from shrimp. Cover seafood with water in a large pot, then add bay leaves, thyme, basil, marjoram, salt, black pepper, and sliced sausage and simmer for 1 hour.

In a second pot, melt butter and sauté the celery, onion, garlic, carrots, and bell pepper for 10 minutes or until brown but not burnt. Remove from the pot and set aside.

Sprinkle 2 tablespoons of flour in the empty pot and brown it in butter. Then, slowly stir in 1 cup of the seafood stock from the simmering pot until the flour turns into a smooth gravy. Stir constantly to prevent lumps from forming.

After gravy is smooth, add the liquid from the first pot into the brown gravy pot, then add the vegetables, seafood, tomatoes, and black-eyed peas, and stir in the hot peppers, parsley, Worcester sauce, and oyster sauce. Let simmer for another 60 minutes. Add more water if it becomes too dry. It should have a loose consistency. Serve warm over rice or on its own.

Storage: This meal can be refrigerated for three days and will keep in the freezer for three months.

. . . .

SPICY SEASONING PEPPER

MAKES ½ CUP

This spicy seasoning can add some heat to your soups or can be used to marinate meat, poultry, and fish.

INGREDIENTS

1 teaspoon coarsely ground black
  pepper
½ teaspoon cayenne pepper
1 teaspoon chili powder
1 teaspoon smoked paprika

1 teaspoon garlic powder
1 teaspoon ground ginger
1 teaspoon salt
½ teaspoon cumin
½ teaspoon cane sugar

DIRECTIONS

Mix all ingredients and store in a labeled glass jar in a cool, dry place.

MAMA SHAFIA'S WARM SALAD

SERVES 3
COOK TIME: 60 MINUTES

Since cold foods are not encouraged in the postpartum period, we warm salad so a new mama can eat it. A warm salad is when all the salad ingredients are warmed in a lightly oiled skillet. This allows new postpartum mothers to indulge in the freshness of a salad without the negative effects of cold, raw food.

INGREDIENTS

1 head romaine lettuce
1 medium tomato, sliced
1 cucumber, sliced
Himalayan salt to taste
Freshly ground black pepper to taste

1 tablespoon toasted sesame oil, plus
  more to coat the skillet
2 teaspoons balsamic vinegar
1 teaspoon honey
1 teaspoon soy sauce

DIRECTIONS

Cut off the bottom of the lettuce head, then rinse every leaf and dry them by laying them on a clean dish towel. Slice the tomato in circles and lay them on a dish towel as well. This helps absorb the excess water from the vegetables. Do the same with the cucumbers. Lightly season all vegetables with a few dashes of Himalayan salt and freshly ground black pepper.

Evenly coat a large cast-iron skillet with toasted sesame oil. There should be about 3 inches of oil in the pan. Wait until the oil is hot, then lay as many lettuce leaves as you can fit into your skillet and warm them for 30 seconds, then flip them over and heat for another 30 seconds. Continue this process until all the vegetables have been heated. Turn the heat off and layer all the vegetables back in the pan in the following order: lettuce on the bottom, then tomatoes, then cucumbers on top.

Put all the warmed ingredients in a bowl and season the salad with two shakes of salt and one shake of black pepper.

Make your dressing: Mix balsamic vinegar, toasted sesame oil, honey, and soy sauce, then warm the mixture up over low heat. Drizzle over salad and serve.

Storage: This cannot be refrigerated or stored.

POSTPARTUM RECUPERATION DRINKS

I always bring mama a cup of tea when I visit, and I often have some myself. Not only are warm beverages important for hydration and health, but sharing a cup of tea is a ritual that celebrates mama and builds in time for you to talk with her about how she's doing.

· ·

WASSAIL TEA

SERVES 6
COOK TIME: 1 HOUR
This drink is traditionally made to be shared with guests. Make this tea when family and friends come to see mama.

INGREDIENTS

5 quarts of water
1 large (6-inch) ginger root, grated
1 (24-ounce) bottle pineapple
  juice
1 (12-ounce) can frozen concentrated
  orange juice

1 (12-ounce) can frozen concentrated
  apple juice
1 (12-ounce) can cranberry juice
1 whole cinnamon stick
½ teaspoon ground cloves
¼ cup granulated raw sugar

DIRECTIONS

Fill a large pot with 4 quarts of water or 3 cans of water per 12 ounces of frozen juice. In a separate pot, boil grated ginger in 2 cups of water for 20 minutes, then let cool. Once cool, strain the ginger and add the liquid back to the large pot of water.

Add pineapple juice, orange juice, apple juice, cranberry juice, cinnamon stick, cloves, and sugar, and simmer for 30 minutes. Remove from heat. Serve hot.

· ·

RELAXING TEA

SERVES 8
The name here says it all: This tea is best for when mama wants to relax. Lemon balm, chamomile, catnip, nettle, and lavender have long been used for their calming properties. Be sure to check with your healthcare provider for any contraindications before taking any herbs.

INGREDIENTS

10 cups water

2 tablespoons dried lemon balm

2 tablespoons dried chamomile

1 teaspoon dried catnip

1 teaspoon dried, food-grade lavender

2 teaspoons dried nettle

5 tablespoons honey

Squeeze of lemon juice

DIRECTIONS

Bring water to a boil, then turn off the heat, add the herbs, and cover. Let steep for 15 minutes. Strain tea into a tea pot or pitcher and add honey. Serve hot or warm, with a squeeze of lemon.

WOMB TEA

SERVES 8

The body is amazing, and during postpartum, it works day and night to return to its pre-pregnancy state. Granny Midwives knew that drinking certain herbal teas would support the body in doing this natural work more effectively. This vitamin-and-mineral-rich tea helps tone the uterus so it can shrink to its pre-pregnancy size.

INGREDIENTS

1 cup grated fresh ginger root

10 cups water

1 tablespoon dried raspberry leaves

1 tablespoon dried chasteberry (vitex)

2 teaspoons dried rosehip

2 tablespoons dried red clover blossom

2 teaspoons spearmint

Organic honey (2 teaspoons per 4-ounce cup)

DIRECTIONS

Boil ginger root in water for 20 minutes, then remove from heat and add the remaining herbs. Cover pot and let steep for 15 minutes. Strain tea into a tea pot or glass pitcher, and add honey according to individual preference. Serve hot or at room temperature.

BREASTMILK TEA

SERVES 6

This tasty recipe contains herbs that help with breastmilk production. As always, check with your healthcare provider when taking herbs to ensure they don't interfere with medications or preexisting conditions.

INGREDIENTS

½ gallon water

2 tablespoons fennel seed

2 tablespoons dried nettle

1 tablespoon dried blessed thistle

2 tablespoons dried vervain

2 teaspoons of fenugreek

Honey to taste

DIRECTIONS

Bring water to a simmer, then turn off heat and immediately add each herb. Cover pot and let steep for 15 minutes, strain, and serve hot or room temperature. Add honey according to individual preference.

EMOTIONAL SUPPORT TEA

SERVES 6

Mama will experience a range of feelings throughout her postpartum period. This emotional support tea, also known as Happy Tea, has herbs that Granny Midwives historically used to encourage a good mood.

INGREDIENTS

8 cups water

2 tablespoons dried spearmint

2 tablespoons dried lemon balm

2 teaspoons dried Gotu Kola

1 teaspoon dried food-grade lavender

5 tablespoons honey or to taste

DIRECTIONS

Bring water to a simmer, then turn off the heat and immediately add the herbs. Cover pot and let steep for 15 minutes. Serve hot or at room temperature. Add honey to taste.

POSTPARTUM DESSERTS

Fresh or stewed fruits were normally served as puddings and considered after-meal desserts. These sweet treats can be traced back to our African ancestors. Desserts are historically made to mark special occasions, like births, marriages, life transitions, and family gatherings.

RICE PUDDING[10]

SERVES 6
COOK TIME: 60 MINUTES

Rice pudding is a testament to African American resilience and resourcefulness. It remains a cherished dish, often associated with warmth, family, and cultural pride. Though an everyday staple, it is also made during special times, like the birth of a new baby. Serve it to a new mother whenever she wants. It works especially well as a morning or midday snack, providing her with energy from the rice, spices, sugar, and eggs.

INGREDIENTS

3 tablespoons butter
2 eggs
½ cup coconut sugar
1 cup cooked rice, preferably a day old
½ cup raisins (optional)
½ teaspoon salt

½ teaspoon vanilla extract
2 cups milk
1 cup heavy cream
1 teaspoon nutmeg
2 dashes ground cinnamon

DIRECTIONS

Preheat oven to 350°F (175°C). Lightly grease a 9 x 9 baking dish with butter.

In a large bowl, mix eggs and sugar together, then add the rice and raisins, if using. Mix well. Next, add salt and vanilla extract. Warm the milk and cream together in a small saucepan, then add in butter to melt. Pour the milk mixture into the rice mixture and combine. Pour mixture into the prepared baking dish. Sprinkle with nutmeg and cinnamon. Place baking dish in a pan of hot water. Set in the oven and bake for 45 to 50 minutes, stirring it after the first 15 minutes. Bake until firm. Serve warm or hot whenever mama wants it.

Storage: Store in the refrigerator for three to seven days or freeze for up to one month.

PEACH COBBLER

SERVES 6
COOK TIME: 60 MINUTES

You can't go wrong with peach cobbler, whether it's for a holiday, Sunday supper, or simply to use up fresh peaches. It's a great fruit dessert for any occasion!

INGREDIENTS

½ cup unsalted butter
1 cup self-rising flour

1 cup coconut sugar
1 cup milk

2 (16-ounce) cans of peaches, drained
½ teaspoon cinnamon

½ teaspoon nutmeg
⅛ teaspoon allspice

DIRECTIONS

Preheat oven to 350°F (175°C).

Melt butter in a baking dish. In a large bowl, mix flour, sugar, and milk until smooth, and pour batter over melted butter. Do not stir.

Using the same bowl, gently combine the peaches with cinnamon, nutmeg, and allspice, then evenly pour the mixture over the batter. Do not stir.

Bake for 45 to 50 minutes until golden brown and bubbly. Let cool for about 10 minutes before serving.

Storage: Store in the refrigerator for three days.

· ·

SWEET POTATO PIE

SERVES 6
COOK TIME: 55 MINUTES

This is an African American staple and an all-time favorite for mamas and their families. Enjoy with a cup of warm tea.

INGREDIENTS

9 medium-sized sweet potatoes, peeled and cubed
2 sticks butter, softened
½ cup cane sugar
½ cup firmly packed dark brown sugar
½ teaspoon salt
¼ teaspoon nutmeg
1 cup flour

3 eggs
⅓ cup fresh orange juice (no pulp)
2 cups milk
1 tablespoon vanilla flavor
2 (9-inch) piecrusts
For two pies: Divide pie filling into separate 9-inch piecrusts

DIRECTIONS

Preheat oven to 350°F (175°C).

Boil the sweet potatoes until soft, then drain.

Combine butter, cane sugar, dark brown sugar, salt, and nutmeg in a large bowl and mix by hand or with an electric mixer until creamy.

Beat in the sweet potatoes and flour until well mixed, then beat in eggs, orange juice, and milk. Add vanilla flavor.

Use about 4 cups of filling per 9-inch piecrust, and bake for 50 to 60 minutes, until potatoes are firm and piecrusts are lightly brown. Let cool and serve.

Storage: Pie can last for three days in the refrigerator.

. . . .

COCONUT CAKE

SERVES 8
COOK TIME: 60 MINUTES

By the early twentieth century, coconut cake had become a staple in Southern Black households, often served at celebrations, church gatherings, and special occasions. Today, coconut cake remains a cornerstone of Southern cuisine, symbolizing resilience, celebration, and the enduring influence of Black cooking. And with a new mama and baby, a coconut cake is always on the menu.[11]

INGREDIENTS

½ cup butter, plus extra for buttering cake pans
2 cups all-purpose flour, sifted, plus extra for flouring cake pans
3 teaspoons baking powder
Salt

1 cup cane sugar
2 egg yolks, beaten
2 teaspoons coconut extract
Lemon juice
1 cup milk
3 egg whites

DIRECTIONS

Preheat oven to 350°F (175°C). Butter two 9-inch cake pans and lightly dust with flour. Shake the pans over the sink to remove excess flour and set aside.

In a large bowl, whisk together flour, baking powder, and salt.

In a separate bowl, place butter and beat until it becomes shiny. Gradually add sugar in small amounts, mixing after each addition. When the sugar has dissolved in the butter, mix in the egg yolks and stir to combine thoroughly.

Add the coconut extract and lemon juice, then stir. Add ¼ of flour mixture and ½ cup of milk and mix together well. Repeat this, adding the flour mixture and milk slowly until everything has been added and is well mixed.

Now, in another small bowl, beat the egg whites with an egg beater until stiff. When they can stand on their own, add them to the mixture and gently fold them in.

Fill the prepared cake pans equally. Bake on the middle rack for 30 minutes. You'll know they're done when the cake shrinks from the side of the cake pan and the cake bounces back from the touch. Take the cakes out of the oven, remove them from the pans, place them on a cooling rack, cover with a clean, light cloth, and let rest for 10 minutes, or until they're cool enough to be frosted.

Coconut Frosting

INGREDIENTS

3 tablespoons boiling water

2 cups powdered sugar

1 stick butter, softened

2 teaspoons vanilla extract

2 cups shredded coconut

DIRECTIONS

Whip together boiling water, powdered sugar, and butter until smooth. Then, add vanilla extract and shredded coconut flakes, and mix. Once the cakes are cool, smooth a layer of frosting on one cake and sit the other cake on top. Add the remaining frosting to the top, then sprinkle on more coconut flakes according to personal preference. This is a rich cake, so serve in small to medium slices.

Storage: This cake has a shelf life of three days in a cake holder or one month when wrapped in cellophane and frozen.

CHAPTER 11

Traditions and Rituals

My Lord, grant that when I enter into something, I enter with truth, and when I depart, I depart with truth, and grant me by your grace authoritative help.

—Surah Al Isra 80, The Night Journey, Holy Quran

A FRIEND ONCE SHARED WITH ME THE FIRST TIME SHE EXPERIENCED African American postpartum rituals. It was after the birth of her firstborn in 1982. She said after she got home from the hospital, her grandmother took a sheet and wrapped her stomach with it.

"Why is grandma doing this?" she asked her mother.

Her mother replied, "It helps flatten your stomach."

"I have never seen that happen before to anyone," my friend said.

At this point, her grandmother, who was still wrapping, spoke up and said, "That's what's wrong with you new mothers, you think you all know everything. I wrapped your momma's stomach after her births, and my momma wrapped my stomach after my births, and her momma wrapped her stomach after she birthed me."

So my friend stopped protesting and let her grandmother continue doing her thing. She said, "Wrapping that sheet so tight she could hardly breathe." When she had her second baby six years later, she followed all of her grandmother's advice.

Some of us are fortunate to remember African American postpartum practices being done in our families, but for those who didn't get to experience these ancestral treasures firsthand, I'm here to share them with you.

African American postpartum care is full of rituals for the physical, mental, and spiritual health of the new mother, her new baby, and the entire community. Rituals are solemn acts that complete the transition to a higher level of self, which includes becoming a mother, regardless of the number of births you have had. We use rituals to commemorate many life phases, like marriage, graduations, death, and birth. For postpartum, it is the way we keep the attention focused on the sacredness of motherhood and the joy of the newborn. Rituals give meaning to actions that lead to growth and a better understanding of a particular transition in life.

The Granny Midwives saw the postpartum period as sacred for many reasons. Birth was considered a spiritual act and having a baby was seen as a gift from God. They recognized that the process of pregnancy and birth, while natural, was also a life-or-death situation, so postpartum rituals were implemented as a safety net for full recovery. They believed, and modern research has confirmed, that the first forty-two days after birth were the most likely time for problems to occur.[1] For this reason, older women insisted that new mothers followed the "guidelines" passed from generation to generation (discussed throughout this book) to reach postpartum wellness, avoid a setback, keep the baby well, and produce an abundance of milk. These rituals extend beyond physical healing in the first forty-two days. We also have naming ceremonies, placenta practices, and rituals for the end of the lying-in period.

As my friend learned, the foundation of African American postpartum traditions and rituals is listening to your elders with an open mind and heart. Learn from their experiences, the good and the bad; it will only make your postpartum experience better. Our elders, including our grandmothers, healers, Granny Midwives, and spiritualists, carry decades of birthing wisdom within them that came across the ocean with our captured African ancestors and emerged from a divine calling on their life. They developed a wealth of traditions that have been passed down through the generations, just like my friend's grandmother who had wrapped her stomach with a sheet. Now, history repeats itself as we return to the traditions, practices, and rituals of our ancestral mothers. Do yourself the honor of seeking the knowledge of African American postpartum traditions and rituals, give thanks when you find them, study them diligently, document them for later use, share them with others, and practice them yourself.

In the following pages, I will take my own advice as I share guidance to help you practice our traditions and rituals for your postpartum well-being.

THE FOUNDATION OF AFRICAN AMERICAN POSTPARTUM RITUALS

You already know much of this from the principles shared so far, but there are six core concepts of our postpartum rituals. The first step is to embrace them in spirit and practice these ceremonies with love.

1. Spirituality: Belief in a higher power. Praying in silence and out loud, call-and-response, healing circles, laying on of hands to soothe new mamas physically and emotionally.

2. Cleanliness, Inside and Out: God made water our source of life; we are born from it. We wash the body to promote healing and protect against infection and the spread of germs, but also to spiritually honor the new mother's transition and create calmness.

3. Environment Matters: In the days of our Granny Midwives, the home was cleansed through a ceremony of sweeping, mopping, dusting, washing sheets, cleaning the mama and baby's clothes, putting salt in the four corners of the home, fumigating with pine needles, planting basil in the front of the house for blessings and protection, painting the shutters indigo blue for protection, and airing out the house. Today, we clean with organic cleaners, burn sage, frankincense, and sandalwood, or use an infuser with essential oils, such as pine oil, lavender, frankincense, tulsi basil, or a pleasant scent of the mother's preference.

4. Mother Warming: This ritual of keeping mama warm after birth is meant to strengthen her immune system, increase oxygen circulation, build her energy for healing, and create a feeling of comfort. When mothers are warm, they feel happier, sleep better, and recover faster. Heat is considered medicine for postpartum healing. It was common for new mothers to keep a scarf on their head, socks on their feet, and wool blankets and quilts over them for warmth. You can also use a thermostat, fireplace, space heaters, heating pads, rice socks, and hot water bottles. Keep the mother's bed away from windows, plug up any drafty doors, and put plastic or heavy drapes over the windows to keep out cold air.

5. Postpartum Beautification: Showers and baths, oiling the skin; offering beautiful, natural-fabric gowns and sleepwear; caring for hair, nails, feet, and toes; taking pictures of mama and baby; and helping mama put on special jewelry and gowns are all key in making her feel beautiful. I always felt special when my sister's friends would henna my feet during my postpartum period, staining them a beautiful burgundy color, help me put on earrings, and wrap my belly in beautiful African cloth to celebrate me as a new mother.

6. Community Support: Community healing is our lineage. As Michael Twitty writes in his book *The Cooking Gene*, "Black healing culture included the community walking along streams to gather fresh watercress to bring to the sick, and they would take shifts to stay and sit with the infirm so that there was always someone to attend their needs."[2] This should be the same for the postpartum mother. Gladys Milton, midwife and author of *Why Not Me?*, said the neighbors would often attend postpartum cleaning and cooking traditions. This neighborly support included bathing and diapering the baby while the mama observed or relaxed. "It sure made us feel good to know we could help somebody that would appreciate it so much."[3]

In the African American postpartum tradition, the father was also included and considered part of aftercare. He had a vital role to play. The Granny Midwife kept him connected to birth and postpartum traditions by empowering him with appreciation, showing him what to cook, and reminding him to keep the house warm so mama can rest and bask in his love.[4]

We need all fathers, siblings, children, grandparents, and community to relearn African American postpartum care so they can provide the deserved and needed support to keep the mother and baby free of illnesses and stresses and get their blessings by being of service.

ORDER OF RITUALS IN THE EARLY POSTPARTUM PERIOD

While all families and circumstances are different, there are a few rituals that should be done in a particular order to promote optimal health and well-being for mother and baby.

1. Immediately After Delivery of Baby: Pray over the mother and baby with a short prayer: "Dear God, thank you for blessing [mother's name] with a safe birth and a beautiful and healthy baby. Amen." If baby is stillborn, we say a prayer of acceptance and strength to help the family navigate this difficult time (more on this later in the chapter).

2. Warmth and Nourishment: Put baby on mama's chest and cover them with a warm blanket to help mama breastfeed in the first hour. Feed mama some coconut chicken curry soup while she holds her baby until she's had enough. After the placenta is birthed, apply a very warm cloth soaked in a hot herbal solution of comfrey, lavender flowers, and rosemary on the vulva area. If the mother has given birth at a hospital, make and freeze her postpartum tea in the last trimester and bring it to the hospital, where it will thaw. Ask the nurse or healthcare provider to warm it up and help apply it, or the mother can apply it using a peri bottle once she is in the recovery room.

3. Cleanse Mother: Perform a ritual wash of warm water, with sesame oil and Florida Water. Florida Water is a fragrant cologne with a long history in spiritual and cultural practices, particularly in African American and Afro-Caribbean traditions. It's often used for cleansing, protection, and ritual work. You can purchase it at most spiritual botanica stores. Help mama wash her face, arms, hands, front side, backside, and lastly, her feet. Keep the room warm while sponging her. Then, dress her in a clean gown for beauty and easy nursing.

4. Ritual Postpartum Bath: The North African postpartum bathing tradition was full of love and prayer—a beautiful, spiritual, and sacred ceremony. The new mother would sit on a small stool, covered with a heavy blanket from head to toe. Under the stool was a bowl of steaming water with healing herbs. The family women would remove the blanket and wash the mother with lavender soaps as they prayed over her out loud. Once she was soaped up, they would rinse her entire body, except her head, with buckets of warm water. They would gently dry her off, put the blanket back over her head and body, put her slippers on, walk her back to her bedroom to dress her in a gown, and put her back in bed. This is very similar to the African American sponge bathing ritual.

5. Massage Mother Regularly: Use warm sesame oil, castor oil drops with coconut oil, or warmed olive oil. Keep the room warm and use only low lights or draw the window shades to keep the room dark. On day one, massage mama's arms, hands, and legs. On day two, massage her back, and repeat the day one massage. On day three, massage her front, including her uterus, breasts, and abdomen. This helps relieve engorged breasts and intestinal gas, stimulate a bowel movement, and keep the uterus firm. On day four, massage her head and neck. On day five, repeat all the steps again. Massage her legs and feet daily. Respect mama's modesty and keep her covered. You can massage her bare skin under a sheet, or you can give the massage over her sheet or her clothes; it is the mama's choice.

6. Belly Wrapping: This ritual should begin on day one and no later than day two. Belly wrapping stabilizes the womb as it shrinks to its original place in the pelvic area, strengthens the back, reduces the discomfort of postpartum cramping, and helps mama's body regain its nonpregnant shape. Belly wrapping also helps mothers feel secure and balanced within themselves. Mothers who have had a cesarean section should have their bellies bound as well. In this case, however, place a soft folded cotton cloth over the incision, then wrap the mother firmly but not tight. African American belly wrapping should not be painful. I'll share instructions on page 249.

7. Pelvic Steaming: On day three, begin this ritual by adding two tablespoons of dried comfrey and rosemary leaves to a pot of boiled steaming water. Place the steaming pot of herbs under a stool or chair with a hole in the middle. Sit on the stool or chair and wrap a cloth around your waist, extending it to the floor. The fabric will trap the steam to contact your pelvic area for healing. Steam for ten to fifteen minutes or less. You decide. The steam should be comfortably warm, not too hot or painful. Drink water during or after pelvic steaming. Steam every few days or weekly. The history of steaming can be found throughout the African Diaspora. Although this is a traditional practice, please check with your healthcare provider.

8. Rest: Mama should stay in bed for the first ten days, when her cervix closes. She can be up for the bathroom, steaming, postpartum baths, belly wrapping, and caring for her baby. During this rest time, she should be fed warm soups and kept warm by wearing a headscarf, having her feet covered, wearing a warm gown, and being covered with blankets. On day ten, she can be ritually helped out of bed by pulling the covers back, helping her sit up on the edge of the bed, giving her a cup of warm tea and something sweet to eat (date, rice pudding, etc.), then walk her to the family room where she can sit with elevated feet and relax. Although she is out of bed, she is still in her lying-in period. Her only job is to lie around the house, breastfeeding, resting, and sleeping.

9. Circle the House: On the forty-second day, we ritually honor the end of the lying-in period by having the mother circle the house. Clockwise, the mother walks around the house, carrying a small cup of water. As she circles the house, she quietly sings a song of gratitude. A family member walks with the mother holding the baby.[5] This ritual begins with the mother putting on a dress that was smoked on the thirty-eighth or thirty-ninth day. Traditionally, the dress was smoked with dried corn husk, pine needles, or dried sage for purification. Today, mothers use their preferences, such as frankincense, myrrh, or sandalwood, to smoke their clothes. After circling the house, the mother drinks the cup of water; this signifies that she has reentered society.

> ### When a Baby Dies
>
> *My heart is heavy for every mother who lost a baby before it was born or shortly thereafter. Even in this difficult situation, I encourage you to practice the postpartum traditions for your health. Grieve your baby with a belly wrap, drink a cup of sage tea to help dry your milk supply, cry into the postpartum soup that will keep you healthy, and rest and sleep to manage the grief that none can feel but you. You still deserve to be supported as your body heals, so tell your caregivers that you need them to give you your postpartum rituals and traditions. And if you have your baby's placenta, bury it separate from or with your baby. I am so sorry you don't have your baby. My prayers will continue for you.*

INSTRUCTIONS FOR POSTPARTUM BELLY WRAPPING

African American postpartum belly wrapping is our ancient tradition. Wrapping the mother's belly or womb area after birth was mandatory for the first forty-two days postpartum, but it was also done up to twelve weeks. The belly wrap should be checked and adjusted as the uterus shrinks back to its pre-pregnancy size and position.

Benefits of Postpartum Belly Wrapping:

- Keeps the womb area warm
- Helps ease involution discomfort

- Strengthens the back
- Grounds the new mother and helps her feel better emotionally
- Improves posture
- Heals abdominal muscles
- Reshapes mother's waist
- Supports the cesarean section incision area
- Feels good

The Wrapping Cloth

Wrapping is easy. It's best when you can be wrapped by someone. Use four to six yards of any 100 percent cotton cloth, as it is stiff, breathable, and will better support the abdominal area. For a larger mother, I use five to six yards of cloth, and for a mama smaller in stature, four to five yards will be enough. The cloth should be about forty-five inches wide. I like to use African cloth for wrapping because the rich colors and patterns connect us to our ancestors, and studies say vibrant colors and intricate patterns positively affect the brain, relaxing the mind and creating happiness. If you can't access an African print, white or blue indigo is a great protective color. Do not use red, as it represents bleeding.[6]

When to Belly Wrap

Belly wrapping can begin on day one. Usually, I belly wrap after the mother has showered, eaten, and slept. If the mama birthed at 8:00 a.m., then she may be wrapped by 6:00 p.m. that same day. If the mother is not sleepy, then I will wrap her two hours after she has eaten.

How to Belly Wrap[7]

1. Have mother stand up and put her hands on the wall in front of her to stabilize her as she's being wrapped.

2. Rub mama's belly with sesame oil or coconut oil. Fold the cloth in half.
3. Stand behind the mother, place the end of the cloth in the middle of her back and then wrap the rest of the cloth around her front. Make sure the cloth covers from her pubic bone to the top of her fundus (top of the uterus). Pull tight as you wrap the cloth around to her back, and keep wrapping tight until all the cloth is used up. Then, tuck the last piece in the wrap itself. This keeps the wrap on and allows mama to take it off independently if she needs to.

Note: The cloth should be tight but not painful. The mother should be able to use the bathroom while wearing her belly wrap, so make sure you don't wrap her hips. The cloth should cover her lower belly and lower back, not the buttocks. Rewrap after each shower or if the wrap becomes loose.

Caesarean Section Belly Wrapping
1. Fold a small white hand towel in thirds and have mother hold it gently over her incision.
2. Wrap her belly over the cloth as instructed.

Note: For Caesarean moms, do not wrap tightly, and check in with the mother often to make sure she does not feel any pain. She will have to be rewrapped every time she changes her incision tape.[8]

RITUALS BEYOND THE LYING-IN PERIOD

Placenta Ritual
Honoring the placenta is important in African American postpartum culture. The placenta is a fetal organ that supports the life of

the unborn baby. Its delivery marks the beginning of the postpartum period. Since it is a part of the baby, we give it an honorable burial.[9]

Twentieth-century African American midwife traditions say to bury the placenta in the backyard or near the house and place a large rock over it to prevent animals from disturbing it and to mark its location. Though consuming the placenta raw or by encapsulation (placentophagy) has become popular in the twenty-first century, placentophagy is not an African/African American postpartum tradition or ritual.

HOW TO BURY THE PLACENTA
Items needed:
- A shovel or large spoon
- A cloth
- Myrrh
- A large rock, heavy piece of wood, or large ceramic planting pot

The placenta is usually buried by someone other than the mother, like the father, another family member, or the midwife. I have helped plenty of fathers choose an area in their yard, place the placenta in the hole, and say a prayer: "God, we thank you for healthy baby and mama. Continue to bless them, and thank you for the important role of the placenta of keeping the baby fed and healthy while she/he lived inside the womb. Amen." If you do not have a yard, you can bury it in a park, a clay pot of dirt, or in a trusted friend or family member's yard. Or you can burn it and bury the ashes.

The Ritual: The placenta should be buried by someone other than the mother as soon as possible. For a hospital birth, you should bury it by day three.

1. Bless the placenta by rinsing it in plain water, orange blossom water, or Florida Water.
2. Wrap in it a cloth, newspaper, or a brown paper bag. Seek to use a natural, biodegradable product.
3. Dig a hole slightly larger than the placenta and at least twelve inches deep.
4. Gently place the wrapped placenta in the hole and use all the dirt dug out to refill the hole completely. Pat the dirt down with shovels or your feet.
5. Place a large rock or heavy object on top of the dirt. Many people later plant a tree over it, but that is optional.
6. If it's winter and the ground is frozen, you can freeze your placenta and bury it when the earth warms.

BURYING THE UMBILICAL CORD

When the cord dries up and falls off, usually between the third and tenth day, it should be given to a family member who will bring it to the placenta site and add it to the grave. As another tradition, the mother can take a clip of the baby's hair, wrap it in a tissue or small piece of napkin, and bury it at the placenta site. Dig down five to seven inches, place the napkin in the hole, and cover it back with the dirt, replacing the rock as the marker. This symbolizes the connection between mother, child, and placenta.

If it is winter, do not disturb the frozen ground until the snow melts and the earth has thawed. In the meantime, you can bury it in a houseplant until spring arrives.

PLACENTA BURIAL VISIT

After the lying-in period, the mother and baby are taken to the placenta site with the family to honor the placenta. I had my first home birth in a first-floor apartment with a backyard. My husband buried the placenta for us right after the birth. Later, when I felt strong, he brought me to the placenta site so I would know where it was and could let my baby son know when he was older.

While you can do as I did and simply visit with your own personal ritual, you can also do the following:

1. Begin with everyone facing the east, which represents where energy rises from every day.
2. Say this three times: *We recognize all that is holy and sacred here today.*
3. Using water from a wooden cup, African calabash, or small clay bowl, pour your libation on the burial site to remember the higher life force and your ancestors.
4. As a final honoring, ask all who are present to call out the names of the ancestors, or honor the site in silence.
5. Lay the baby down on her placenta site for reconnection and to be humble growing up.

North African Closing the Bones

Although I am sharing this with you, as it is an important postpartum ritual, please note that *this must be performed by someone trained in the practice.* It is a skill that family members were traditionally trained to do. And you can relearn with midwives and doulas who can perform this ritual properly. This ritual generally happens on the fortieth day of the lying-in period to help the mother's bones and organs return to their right position.

In this ritual, mama is given a ritual bath and massaged. Then, the two women who are knowledgeable on this tradition help the mother lay down on a heavy blanket or yoga mat on the floor. The women put a five-yard-long cloth under the mother's hips. Each person picks up an end of the cloth and passes it over to the other person to exchange ends, then they pull the cloth together, down toward the floor, squeezing the mother's hips for a count of sixty-one hundred. When done, they move the cloth up to her pelvic area and repeat the process. This is done for each area of the body until they get to her shoulders. Then, they move back down again, pulling at each point all the way back down to her hips.

When the ritual is complete, mama is fed a cup of warm buttermilk with molasses and a small piece of cornbread and is encouraged to take a nap. The closing of the bones is nurturing and loving because the squeezing is said to represent being hugged. Additionally, the people closing the mother are usually saying silent or audible prayers or singing. Many mothers cry during this ritual, as it creates a healthy emotional release.

Baby-Naming Ceremony

There are many ceremonies and celebrations, like the Christian Baptism and Islamic Akika, that invite extended family and close friends to meet the baby, learn their name, pray for them, congratulate the mother and father, and offer gifts for the baby. This is the same in African American postpartum tradition. These celebrations for new mothers and baby included plenty of sweets, meats, special dishes, and gifts for mama and baby. Mamas wear beautiful clothes to stand out as the new mother. The baby also wears special clothes. The family is responsible for hosting the naming ceremony with celebratory food to thank the Creator for a healthy baby and mother. This is a time of prayer, celebration, singing, and dancing may be involved, for gratitude and health. In African culture, there is much honor, love, and prayers for the new mother and her baby during the naming ceremony. It serves as a coming out party, and happens after the lying-in period has ended. I had naming ceremonies for most of my babies. We had plenty of food, drumming, prayers, and a beautiful time honoring me as a new mother and meeting my new baby. I know my oxytocin soared, I was so happy showing off my baby.

NEWBORN CARE

I learned newborn care by watching my mother care for my infant niece. She massaged after her bath, using warm vegetable oil. She laid my niece on a folded towel, massaging her legs, arms, back, and stomach areas. My mother massaged her face, and told me that you have to shape her head to make it round. After the end of the massage, she would do an inverision on my niece. Interesting, my niece never cried. It was exciting when I travel to Senegal, and observed the mothers massaging their babies in a similar fashion as my mother. How did my mother know this, it must have been passed down through generations. African massage is a sophisticated method for proper infant development, ending with infant inversion as well. Later in the '90s, infant massage became popular, and people began studying East Indian infant massage. I was grateful that I learned African infant massage from my mama, and I practiced it on my seven children being sure to shape their heads, as mother taught me, and what was reinforced on my trip to Senegal. I learned that baby massage, head shaping, and inversion has long existed in Africa as a common tradition and as an act of duty, love, and infant development. My husband says he loves my round head, and I have to thank my mother for that.

It is a myth that we spoil babies by responding to their cries. Your baby can only communicate by crying. So don't ignore the crying baby. Pick up your baby, feed, change, bath, or rock gently and sing them to calmness. African-centered newborn care means that we respond immediately to their cries. This teaches our babies that they are seen and safe. If they keep crying, try a full warm bath that covers the shoulders, with low lighting for babies who tend be fussy. Water is medicinal, and babies grew in warm amniotic fluid for nine months, so a warm bath can calm them.

There are many traditions around cord care, such as using drying herbs as well as using white vinegar to wipe the base of the cord, to speed up drying. The good news is the navel cord has no nerves and therefore it is painless for the baby. The most important thing is to help it dry so that it can fall off quickly. Keep the diaper folded under the cord so that it can air dry, and don't let wet diapers touch the cord. Check with your provider for support.

It's important that we dress our babies according to the weather, and according to the way you dress that day. If it is cold and you are wearing socks, a coat and a hat, dress your baby the same way. And if it is hot and you are wearing light material clothes, dress the baby the same way, in light cotton clothes with light socks. The sun strength affects a baby's skin differently, so keep them protected from the sun during the hottest time of day, and only let them get intermittent sun rays on their skin. There is a new trend to bring babies out without hats and socks during cold weather. Granny Midwife would say, dress that baby warm. Remember cold weather weakens the immune system. Baby can't talk, so we have to be sensitive to their needs. This is the core of newborn care.

CHAPTER 12

Improving Pregnancy Outcomes for Black Women

Dear God, hear my prayer and accept it. Anoint this mother with the spirit of compassion, self-confidence, and faith. Keep her from harm's way, and keep harm's way from her. Let the light of protection surround her. Grant her the knowing to know what is best for her.

I pray that her family and healthcare providers commit to giving her the best care for full postpartum recuperation, guidance from you, and acknowledging this sacred time of new motherhood with all the things necessary to bring forth health, happiness, and abundance. Amen.

A S A BLACK WOMAN WHO HAS BEEN PREGNANT THIRTEEN TIMES AND birthed seven healthy, full-term babies, the first six of whom were born at home and the last born at the hospital, I am promoting what I know to be true, not only as a trusted and skilled midwife, but as a woman who has trusted my body, my wisdom, and the Creator to lead me in my pregnancies and postpartum journeys. I stand in spirit and solidarity with the hundreds of thousands of Black women who have birthed safely.

It makes sense to expect low maternal mortality in the United States, as it is a high-income country with state-of-the-art medical technology, but in reality, the United States has the highest maternal mortality rate of all high-income countries.[1] This is true regardless of race, but we know that Black women disproportionately experience higher rates of both maternal mortality and morbidity, regardless of their educational, marital, or economic status.

Research is unveiling what we already know: Systemic racism and implicit bias are at the root of increased Black maternal mortality, which can take place at any part of the pregnancy/postpartum cycle. In 2020, the numbers regarding Black maternal mortality looked like this: 25.7 percent of fatalities occurred during pregnancy; 11.1 percent happened on the day of delivery; 16.2 percent happened on days one through six postpartum; 20.2 percent took place between seven to forty-two days postpartum; and 26.9 percent died between forty-two days to one year. This is unacceptable and unnecessary, as 60 percent of poor outcomes are preventable.[2]

As we know, this increased mortality rate is the result of a medical system that does not listen to Black women and disregards our symptoms. It is also the result of long-standing, racist social determinants, like food deserts and environmental contaminants. Addressing these challenges requires a multifaceted approach aimed at dismantling the barriers that prevent Black women from receiving the maternal care they need and deserve, like adequate access to culturally competent and quality prenatal care, geographical accessibility, comprehensive insurance, community based care, in areas where the closest institution for maternity care is within reach in thirty minutes by public transportation. All of these deficits are linked to systemic racism, in which the Black community is herded and corralled into areas that are lacking in resources that create an organic quality of life, such as quality food, safety, housing, education, child-friendly recreational opportunities, and public transportation.

> ## Maternal Mortality Causes[3]
>
> *The causes of maternal mortality are numerous, but the most common ones include ectopic pregnancy, cardiovascular disease, sepsis, obstetrical hemorrhage, preeclampsia/eclampsia/hypertensive disorders, cesarean deliveries, venous thromboembolism, amniotic fluid embolism, unaddressed medical concerns, and systemic racism.*
>
> ### Key Facts
>
> - *Every ninety seconds, a woman dies during childbirth; most of these deaths are preventable.*
> - *The most significant causes of Black maternal mortality are hemorrhage and preeclampsia.*
> - *Maternal mortality is higher among African American women because of implicit bias and systemic racism.*
> - *Skilled care before, during, and after childbirth can save the lives of women and newborn babies.*
> - *As part of the United Nations's Sustainable Development Goals, the target is to reduce the global maternal mortality ratio to less than 70 deaths per 100,000 live births between 2016 and 2030. The United States did not meet the 2015 Sustainable Development Goals.*
> - ***Bias and Discrimination:*** *Racial bias and discrimination in the healthcare system can lead to Black women's concerns being minimized or dismissed, contributing to delays in diagnosis and treatment.*

- *Social Determinants of Health:* Factors influenced by systemic racism, such as lack of housing, poor educational opportunities, and economic instability affect Black women's health and well-being, impacting their pregnancy childbirth and mothering experiences.
- *Underlying Health Conditions:* Higher rates of hypertension and diabetes among Black women can increase pregnancy-related risks, necessitating more sensitive and comprehensive perinatal care.

HOW TO REDUCE MATERNAL MORTALITY

The medical system can reduce Black maternal mortality by mandating respectful, high-quality care, addressing systemic biases, and ensuring timely intervention for urgent maternal warning signs. We need a national shift that centers women by creating policies that give them a strong start at birth, like access to quality food and more Black midwives for home births, birth centers, and hospitals. My vision has always been to have a Black midwife every ten blocks. We need easy access to early and quality prenatal care with healthcare professionals who welcome and respect Black women and our families and listen when we say something is wrong and act.[4]

The Importance of Informed Consent

Informed consent is a legal and ethical obligation for medical practitioners in the United States to make sure patients are informed before a medical procedure. It is a central aspect of patient-centered care and safety that should translate to better birth outcomes. If your provider is not practicing informed consent, report them to the president of the hospital and seek another doctor.

The Foundations of Informed Consent:

Communication: *A healthcare provider educates the patient on the medical procedure, including the risks, benefits, and alternatives.*

Understanding: *The provider assesses the patient's understanding of the information, using the patient's language.*

Decision: *The patient makes a decision about whether to proceed with the procedure or not, and is respected by the medical team, regardless of their decision.*

Documentation: *The provider documents the process in the patient's medical records, including their understanding of the information and their preferences.*

TAKE ACTION FOR A POSITIVE BIRTH EXPERIENCE

Racial discrimination can create an excess of stress hormones for Black women who experience it regularly, which can negatively affect their general and reproductive health and cause premature labor and birth, high blood pressure, and depression. As Black women, there are things we can do to counteract our body's responses to stress and support our mental, physical, and reproductive health.

Things to Acknowledge and Remember:

- There is nothing wrong with your skin color.
- Write a birth plan to document and share your goals for your birth and postpartum experience.
- You are entitled to your feelings.
- Be kind to yourself.
- Meditate, get massages, and drink plenty of water.
- Write the mantra on page xvi, place it on your refrigerator, your bedroom and bathroom mirror. Say it five time per day, believe it, because it is true.
- Read self-help books by Black female authors. Here are a few options:

  * *One Day My Soul Just Opened Up* by Iyanla Vanzant—A guided journal that helps readers process emotions and find inner peace
  * *What I Know For Sure* by Oprah Winfrey—A collection of reflections on joy, resilience, and gratitude
  * *Year of Yes* by Shonda Rhimes—Encourages readers to step out of their comfort zone and embrace life fully
  * *The Black Girl's Guide to Self-Care* by Kristin D. Hemingway—A thirty-day workbook focused on self-care practices
  * *365 Affirmations for Black Women* by Mia Harper—Daily affirmations to boost confidence and self-love
  * *Self-Care for Black Women* by Layla Moon—A mental health workbook designed to quiet inner criticism and promote self-esteem

NUTRITIONAL HEALTH

Preconception health is a must for both the woman and the man. Here are some things you can do to optimize your health before pregnancy:

- Enter pregnancy as close as possible to your ideal weight. It's okay to be five pounds over or under.
- Use the African Diet Heritage food pyramid as your nutritional guide.[5]
- Eat three cups of dark leafy vegetables daily to prevent anemia.
- Eat seventy-five ounces of protein daily.
- Walk thirty minutes per day, rain or shine.
- Drink at least seven eight-ounce cups of water daily.
- Drink a cup of red raspberry leaf, ginger, and nettle tea each day. Use one teaspoon of each herb to two cups of boiled water. Cover cup and let steep for ten to fifteen minutes.

MINDSET

1. Don't fear pregnancy or growing your baby. Realize that growing and birthing a child is an ancient practice that women experience worldwide. Fear adds undue stress and can lead to poor decision-making and health outcomes. Educate yourself. Enjoy your pregnancy! Black women have the right to have children where and when we please, and a provider of our choice.

2. Build your birth team. The members of your birth team can include family, a midwife, birth doula, lactation consultant, childbirth educator, and postpartum doula. It's important that you find a Black midwife you love and trust and who respects the father/partner, as mothers who hire midwives are more likely to have better birth outcomes.[6] Additionally, it's a good idea to invest in a Black doula who will advocate for you, support your healthy lifestyle, help you and your partner enjoy the pregnancy, and be prepared for birth and postpartum. Doula care reduces cesarean sections and medical interventions, decreases the use of regional anesthesia, increases breastfeeding rates in the first hour post birth, and promotes mother satisfaction with their birth experience.[7] Your birth team should be your cheerleader, listening to your needs and giving you confidence in your abilities. They should be a partner in your perinatal care.

3. Choose a hospital that will respect your rights and wishes. Use the Irth app to find where Black women are having positive birth experiences.

4. Refer to yourself as a health consumer, not a "patient," because pregnancy is not an illness. You have the right to choose a team of providers that supports you and makes you feel safe.

5. Take childbirth education classes and read *The Doula Guide to Birth* by Ananada Lowe and Rachel Zimmerman and *Safe in a Midwife's Hands* by Linda Janet Holmes. Take a breastfeeding workshop before you become pregnant or by the second trimester of pregnancy. Reading and taking classes are essential to know what to expect and to visualize how you want your baby to enter the world.

6. Create your birth vision. Black women must have faith in God and believe in their bodies to carry and birth a baby. Celebrate motherhood and practice the African American postpartum traditions and recipes I've shared throughout the book.

De-stressing Practices

- Take three deep breaths in through nose, expand the belly, and exhale through the mouth. Then listen to your heartbeat and remember that you know your body better than anyone else. You know how you feel, no matter what the machines or the medical system says. The baby lives in you.

- Each day, write about how you are feeling. What feels different? What are you concerned about? What feels good and why?
- Remind yourself that it's your human right to receive quality health care. Bring your spouse, partners, family members, doulas, and friends to your prenatal visits for emotional support and advocacy.
- Take a daily walk for at least ten minutes. Walk barefoot in the grass, when possible. Sunbathe for vitamin D.
- Have fun!
- During pregnancy, rest on your left side for five to ten minutes each day without reaching for your phone.
- Get a counselor to help reduce stress.

Do not apologize for being vigilant about protecting your health and life. Let your healthcare provider know that you are aware of the Black maternal mortality rate, and you want them to tell you how they will protect your life during your perinatal experience. If you don't get a satisfactory answer, report them on Irth, write a letter to your insurance company, send a copy to the head of the hospital, and save a copy for your records. You deserve quality care and support for your self-advocacy. If your healthcare provider is not supportive, change doctors or hospitals, then file a formal complaint. These recommendations carry over to the health of your baby; too many Black babies die before reaching their first birthday, which most often is also preventable.

PROTECT YOUR MATERNAL HEALTH CHECKLIST

Nutritional Support

- ❏ Preconception health is a must.
- ❏ Heal your anemia before you conceive.
- ❏ Get a full bloodwork panel to check the following numbers:
  - ○ Hemoglobin
  - ○ Serum iron
  - ○ Ferritin iron stores
  - ○ Blood sugar

- ❏ Consume at least ninety grams of protein per day during pregnancy and post-partum.
- ❏ Take quality prenatal vitamins, including iron and vitamin C with your meals. As always, check with your healthcare provider before taking any supplements.
- ❏ Gain twenty-five to thirty-five pounds during pregnancy—more if you're under twenty-one years old or underweight, and less if you're overweight. Let your healthcare provider guide you.
- ❏ Eat the recipes in this book for healthy postpartum recuperation. All of the soups can also be eaten when pregnant.
- ❏ Drink at least seven cups of water daily.
- ❏ Drink a cup of red raspberry, ginger, and nettle tea daily.

Health Care

- ❏ Employ a Black midwife or African American obstetrician.
- ❏ Get a complete physical to rule out any illness.
- ❏ Begin prenatal care early and attend all of your appointments.
- ❏ Purchase a blood pressure cuff to monitor your blood pressure in between visits. If you have a blood pressure over 120/80, call your healthcare provider.
- ❏ Talk to a healthcare provider if anything feels wrong or concerning.
- ❏ Ask if you need low-dose aspirin to prevent preeclampsia.
- ❏ Insist that your medical provider listen to you, and if they don't, request a patient advocate and write the president of the hospital.
- ❏ Share your pregnancy history during each medical care visit for up to one year after delivery.
- ❏ Connect with healthcare and social support systems before, during, and after pregnancy.

- ❑ Take prescribed medication on time.
- ❑ Count the kicks of your unborn baby.
- ❑ Know the signs of premature labor, and get help right away if anything feels concerning.

At-Home Support

- ❑ Take a ten-minute walk twice daily (thirty minutes a day is best).
- ❑ Have fun—watch comedy or listen to positive music.
- ❑ Eat protein and vegetables.
- ❑ Eat when you are hungry.
- ❑ Keep oranges to snack on.
- ❑ Rest on your left side for five to fifteen minutes daily.
- ❑ Absolutely no:

  - ○ Bad news, on TV or online
  - ○ Secondhand smoke
  - ○ Alcohol
  - ○ Illegal drugs or marijuana
  - ○ Physical or emotional violence or abuse

Postpartum Period

- ❑ Lie-in for six weeks after the birth of your baby.
- ❑ Breastfeed for at least thirteen months for maternal and infant health benefits.
- ❑ Ask for help from friends and family.
- ❑ Keep your stress levels low to prevent postpartum health problems.

Dangerous Symptoms

- ❑ Go to the hospital if you experience any of these symptoms as they could indicate a potentially life-threatening complication:

  - ○ Increase in blood pressure
  - ○ Severe headache
  - ○ Extreme swelling of hands, face, or legs
  - ○ Spots in your vision
  - ○ Difficulty breathing
  - ○ Heavy vaginal bleeding or discharge
  - ○ Fever
  - ○ Overwhelming fatigue or a general feeling of being unwell

PRACTICE OUR TRADITIONAL WAYS FOR
POSTPARTUM HEALTH

For every maternal death, one hundred women experience some level of postpartum health issues, known as "maternal morbidity." Low-level issues are referred to as normal discomfort, and severe maternal morbidities are referred to as "near misses," when pregnant women nearly die in childbirth. And because more Black women are dying from preventable causes in childbirth than ever before, that means more Black women are suffering from maternal morbidity.

I bring attention to this serious issue because it is not talked about enough. When a mother has experienced a traumatic birth experience or is ill during her postpartum period for any reason, families are often unaware that she needs additional support. When you are ill after your birth, your body will use your energy to heal itself, reducing the amount of energy you'll have to care for yourself and your newborn. It will be difficult for you to enjoy and care for your baby if you're not feeling well. You will need more help, and that's okay.

Let your husband, partner, family, and close friends know the truth about your health, and ask them for help. Be specific by saying something, like "The doctors said I lost too much blood during/after my birth, so I will be feeling weak for months until my iron increases. Can you come by once a day for an hour or two to help me with the baby/warm up food/bring me meals/put my vitamins on my plate/keep my bathroom, kitchen, or bedroom clean/drive me to my doctor visits, etc. Make a list of tasks that will help you heal and reduce your stress during your postpartum period.

It is common for a new mother to experience discomfort after her baby's birth, and this discomfort can vary depending on her individual pain threshold, the type of birth she had, the number of times she has given birth, and the level of support she has postpartum. Though some women experience minimal discomfort after they have a baby, every woman's body will need to recuperate internally from pregnancy and birth.

All of these factors highlight why we must practice African American postpartum traditions. The first forty-two days are when mama's health issues are most noticeable. Too often, low-level maternal morbidities are normalized as part of the postpartum period, so mothers are told to "wait it out" or that their symptoms will resolve themselves over time. This does not address the underlying problem, causing many maternal morbidities to linger longer after the birth than they should.

Low-Level Postpartum Illness

Low-level maternal morbidities come in all forms, including:

- Backaches
- Burning on urination
- Constipation
- Cracked nipples
- Fatigue
- Headaches
- Mastitis
- Perineal or pelvic pain
- Depression
- Hemorrhaging
- Hemorrhoids
- Infections (uterine and incision)
- Iron anemia
- Postpartum-induced hypertension (PIH)
- Prolapsed uterus
- Urinary incontinence
- Uterine inversion

It is important to know that without relief, low-level morbidities can worsen and affect the physical and mental well-being of postpartum mothers. Know your body, learn the warning signs, and seek immediate treatment. If needed, go to the emergency room, call an ambulance, and contact your healthcare provider. Follow the traditions and rituals I have shared in this book as they are the best way to achieve and sustain wellness after birth. Our African American postpartum traditions bring relief and healing during this time when discomforts and pain are common.[8]

Focus on Preventing or Healing Anemia

Pregnancy-related anemia, if left untreated, will become postpartum anemia, which is a serious maternal health issue.[9] Many mothers are discharged from the hospital without being checked for anemia, yet studies suggest that most mothers are anemic on discharge, particularly if they were anemic while pregnant. Anemia in the postpartum period is responsible for headaches, shortness of breath, depression, exhaustion, cold hands and feet, pale skin or pallor, and overall weakness.

Once I became a midwife, I learned the seriousness of anemia. I remember an elder woman saying, "She has low blood." At the time, I did not know what that meant, but I noticed that the Granny Midwives were always cooking liver and encouraging new mothers to eat it to avoid "low blood" or anemia. In my doula trainings with groups of twenty to twenty-five Black women, I began asking who was currently anemic, and every time, at least a quarter of the room would raise their hands.

Anemia is a severe health problem for Black women because we have a higher risk of anemia in pregnancy, which is related to maternal and fetal/neonatal complications.[10] Maternal exhaustion is not usual and, many times, is a result of postpartum anemia. Normal hemoglobin and red blood cell count is essential for a new mother to obtain wellness in her postpartum period to have the emotional and physical strength to care for herself and her newborn. Between 2011 and 2020, there was more than a 100 percent increase in anemia prevalence in African American patients.[11] Because of this, additional research has identified the need for community health interventions on anemia among African American pregnant women.

Being anemic at the time of delivery creates unnecessary risks for postpartum hemorrhaging and shock due to blood loss, which can cause ongoing postpartum health issues for new mamas.

Preventing and Treating Anemia

You can reduce your chances of developing postpartum issues by being in your best health before you get pregnant. If you have anemia, cure it before becoming pregnant. The following foods are iron rich, so try to eat them before you try to conceive, even if you don't like them:

- *Chicken livers (eat twice a week)*
- *Collard greens, turnip greens, and spinach (eat daily)*
- *Navy, red, and black beans cooked in a true cast-iron pot*
- *Eat foods high in vitamin C with iron-rich vegetables. For example, drink lemon water while eating your greens, or eat bell peppers with your greens. This will help your body absorb the iron better.*
- *Refrain from drinking black tea, coffee, wine, or beer, or consuming foods with tannic acid (like grapes, pomegranates, chocolate, etc.) close to when you eat iron-rich*

foods. Tannic acid tends to block the absorption of iron in the body.

- *Take a low-dose iron tablet with food and according to the directions.*

Remember to ask your medical provider to check your iron and provide support to help you reach normal levels.

Postpartum:

- *Eat a protein- and iron-rich diet filled with vitamin-fortified foods to recuperate and regain your strength within a healthy amount of time.*
- *Ask your healthcare provider to check your hemoglobin level before you are discharged from the hospital. If needed, follow up at four and twenty-six weeks.[12]*
- *Try to continue breastfeeding for thirteen months, as breastfeeding often delays the menstrual cycle, which allows women to rebuild their iron stores from pregnancy and birth.*

MY CLOSING MESSAGE

Black mama, you are a queen. You are brilliant and beautiful. You have experienced a miracle; you have birthed a life. Please take it slow for your reproductive organs to return to their prepregnant state and as you learn motherhood and your newborn. Once you feel ready, celebrate yourself for all that you have achieved, regardless of how you birthed. And for the mamas who lost a baby, you still must observe the lying-in period. You deserve time to grieve and let others care for you in the African American traditional way.

Every woman's postpartum experience is unique to her, so don't compare yourself. Dance to your own rhythm of postpartum recuperation and follow the guidance of the Granny Midwives. They told us to slow down and not rush. They wanted us to stay put, to rest, and to quiet our minds. They said, "Don't worry, have faith, things are going to work out," and I am here to say the same. Relax and enjoy this short window in time. Be comfortable being at the center because you earned it. And keep your faith.

Take care of yourself so you can live a long, full life with your children. You are important to many. Your postpartum care is an investment in your future. You have gifted the world with life, so honor yourself and the Creator with health and rest.

Our ancestors left us their legacy to follow, they gave us the way to be well, and they shared their wisdom so we would know what to do and be able to honor our motherhood crown. We must respect this wisdom and follow through to the best of our ability. This is their love for us.

Love,
Mama Shafia Monroe

Glossary

African American Belly Wrapping: Where a new mother's abdomen is wrapped tightly with cloth to support healing after childbearing.

African Diaspora: The worldwide communities of people of African descent who live outside the African continent.

Cesarean section (C-section): A surgical procedure where a baby is delivered through an incision in the mother's abdomen and uterus. It's often performed when a vaginal delivery would pose a risk to the mother or baby, or when labor complications arise.

Colic: A condition where an otherwise healthy infant experiences frequent, prolonged, and intense crying or fussiness for no apparent reason. It typically follows the "rule of threes"—crying for more than three hours a day, at least three days a week, for more than three weeks.

Doula: A trained professional (usually a woman) who provides emotional support to pregnant, laboring, birthing, and postpartum women.

Engorgement: The swelling or overfilling of a body part with fluid, often blood or lymph. In a postpartum context, it describes breast engorgement, which happens when the breasts become overly full of milk, leading to pain, swelling, and firmness, especially in the early postpartum period.

Episiotomy: A surgical cut (incision) made in the perineum, the area between the vagina and anus, during childbirth to enlarge the vaginal opening.

Fundus: The top part of the uterus, opposite the cervix; the base or bottom of an organ or cavity. It is the part of the organ that is farthest from its opening.

Granny Midwife: African American women who provided midwifery services, particularly in the rural South, until the late 1930s. They were not only skilled in childbirth but also served as community healers, counselors, and advocates for mothers and families.

Heme Iron: Easily absorbable iron found in animal meat.

Hemorrhage: An escape of blood from a ruptured blood vessel, especially when profuse.

Herbal Compress: A cloth soaked in a herbal infusion and applied to the skin for therapeutic purposes. It's a traditional method of delivering herbal remedies to the body, and is often used for pain relief, inflammation, and muscular tension.

Herbs: Vascular plants that have no persistent woody stems aboveground.

Informed Consent: When a doctor shares the possible risks and benefits of a treatment to a patient before they make a health decision.

Involution: The natural shrinking or return of an organ to its normal size, such as the uterus contracting after childbirth.

Iron-Deficient Anemia: A condition characterized by a lack of healthy red blood cells, or hemoglobin.

Laying on of hands: The transmission of healing or spiritual power by a person laying their hands on an ill person.

Lochia: Normal discharge from the uterus after childbirth.

Lying-in Period: The first six weeks of the postpartum period when a new mother rests and is cared for.

Midwife: A trained professional who assists women during pregnancy, childbirth, and postpartum and provides general feminine wellness care. The term comes from Middle English, meaning "with-woman," reflecting their role in supporting birthing individuals.

Motherwit: A deeply rooted concept in African American culture referring to the instinctive wisdom, resilience, and practical intelligence passed down through generations, especially among Black women.

Perineum: The area of the body between the anus and the vulva in females.

Placenta: An organ that forms in the womb (uterus) during pregnancy. The placenta is connected to a developing baby by a tubelike structure called the umbilical cord. Through the umbilical cord, the placenta provides oxygen and nutrients to a developing baby.

Pot Likker/Pot Liquor: The nutrient-rich broth left behind after boiling leafy greens. It's packed with vitamins and minerals, including iron, vitamin A, vitamin C, and vitamin K.

Preeclampsia: A serious pregnancy complication characterized by high blood pressure and protein in the urine, typically occurring after twenty weeks of pregnancy.

Protein: A vital macronutrient made up of long chains of amino acids. It plays a crucial role in building and repairing tissues, supporting immune function, and producing enzymes and hormones. Proteins are found in both animal and plant sources, including meat, fish, eggs, beans, nuts, and legumes.

Setback: When a healthy postpartum mother becomes sick from doing too much too soon.

Social Determinants: The nonmedical factors that influence a person's health and well-being. They include the conditions in which people are born, grow, live, work, and age, as well as the wider forces that shape these conditions.

Vulva: The external female genital organs. The vulva includes the inner and outer lips of the vagina, the clitoris, the opening of the vagina and its glands, the opening of the urethra, and the mons pubis (the rounded area in front of the pubic bone that becomes covered with hair at puberty).

Waiting on: The act of attending to someone.

Preventing Burnout
for Caregivers

THE BEST EXAMPLE WE CAN GIVE A NEW MOTHER IS TO DEMON-strate how we take care of ourselves while caring for her and her newborn. Actions speak louder than words. In African American culture, caregiving is considered healing and spiritual work. Caring for the new mother and newborn is viewed as a blessing. It is energy work because we are helping to restore the mother and because we are dealing with the innocence of a new life. Know that even a little help is appreciated, so do what you can with a good attitude, and don't be overwhelmed.

Steps to Prevent Burnout

- Adjust your attitude.
- Willingly offer postpartum care to the new mother and her family.
- Be of sound mind and health.
- Believe in African American postpartum care.
- Leave your home with a prayer.
- Enter the family's home with a prayer.
- Get rest.
- Eat healthy.

Communal postpartum care is fun because the work is distributed among more than one person. Everyone does something to help, so no one should feel burned out or overwhelmed. There may be circumstances where you are the only one available to offer postpartum care. When this is the case, analyze what resources are available.

Communal Postpartum Care

- Delegate: Ask family members, including children and friends, to help.
- Hire a doula or student doula.
- Hire a midwife or student midwife.
- Create a list of things that need to be done, then share it with family and friends.
- Ask them to choose what they will do and when.

Self-Care Tips

- When cooking for the mama, make enough food for you to eat.
- When you serve her tea, sit and have a cup with her.
- Before entering the house, take a walk around the block.
- When leaving the house, take a walk around the block.
- Wear comfortable clothes when helping.
- Dance to your favorite music.
- Drink a cup of caffeine, Gota Kola and green tea, an hour before offering postpartum care.
- Stay hydrated. This can sometimes increase energy.
- Get seven to nine hours of sleep.
- Remember that your work is a blessing.

Postpartum Recuperation

Sore muscles
- Jaws
- Neck
- Arms
- Legs

Thyroid
- Postpartum thyroiditis

Breasts
- Engorgement
- Tender
- Leaking milk
- Mastitis

Nipples
- Sore
- Cracked
- Raw
- Bleeding

Vulva
- Urethra sore, stinging
- Vagina sore, swollen, puffy

Perineum
- Swelling
- Tears
- Episiotomy stitches

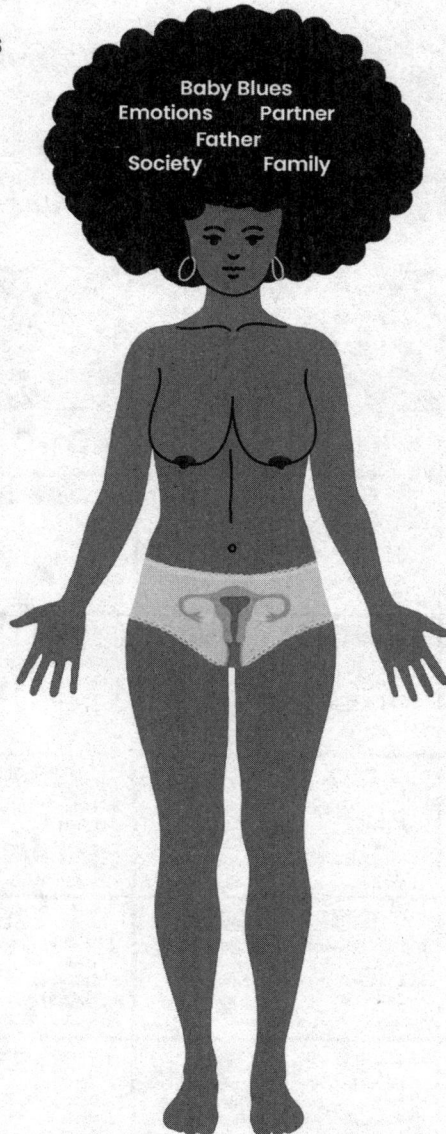

Baby Blues
Emotions   Partner
Father
Society   Family

Cesarean
- Incision soreness
- Urethral catheter
- Uterus
- Involution takes 6–8 weeks
- Cervix takes 10 days to close
- After pains (cramps)

Lochia
- Rubra
- Serosa
- Alba

Lower back
- Sacrum
- Coccyx

Elimination
- Rectum swollen
- Hemorrhoids
- Constipation

Other
- Hair loss
- Thirst
- Hunger
- Sweating

POSTPARTUM RITUAL
- Postpartum blessing • Sitz bath • Yoni steaming • Soups, stews
- Belly binding • Baths • Body massage • Herbal teas

The postpartum recuperation image shows the changes a female body undergoes after giving birth. Postpartum discomforts may be experienced simultaneously, as a few symptoms, or in various combinations over time.

Cervix Closes	10 days
Uterus Shrinks	42 days
Placenta Heals	42 days

POSTPARTUM CARE CALENDAR

42 DAY LYING-IN

Sun	Mon	Tue	Wed	Thu	Fri	Sat
DAY 1 1. Baby Born 2. Rest 3. Warm Stews 4. Sleep	**DAY 2** 1. Belly Wrapping 2. Herbal Sitz Baths 3. Herbal Drinks 4. Soups 5. Shower	**DAY 3** 1. Mom Massage 2. Meals 3. Errands 4. Social Hour Name: ___	**DAY 4** 1. Mom Massage 2. Meals 3. Errands 4. Social Hour Name: ___	**DAY 5** 1. Mom Massage 2. Meals 3. Errands 4. Social Hour Name: ___	**DAY 6** 1. Mom Massage 2. Meals 3. Errands 4. Social Hour Name: ___	**DAY 7** 1. Mom Massage 2. Meals 3. Errands 4. Social Hour Name: ___
DAY 8 1. Mom Massage 2. Meals 3. Errands 4. Social Hour Name: ___	**DAY 9** 1. Mom Massage 2. Meals 3. Errands 4. Social Hour Name: ___	**DAY 10** Cervix Healed +/-	**DAY 11** 1. Mom Massage 2. Meals 3. Errands 4. Social Hour Name: ___	**DAY 12** 1. Mom Massage 2. Meals 3. Errands 4. Social Hour Name: ___	**DAY 13** 1. Mom Massage 2. Meals 3. Errands 4. Social Hour Name: ___	**DAY 14** 1. Mom Massage 2. Meals 3. Errands 4. Social Hour Name: ___
DAY 15 1. Mom Massage 2. Meals 3. Errands 4. Social Hour Name: ___	**DAY 16** 1. Mom Massage 2. Meals 3. Errands 4. Social Hour Name: ___	**DAY 17** 1. Mom Massage 2. Meals 3. Errands 4. Social Hour Name: ___	**DAY 18** 1. Mom Massage 2. Meals 3. Errands 4. Social Hour Name: ___	**DAY 19** 1. Mom Massage 2. Meals 3. Errands 4. Social Hour Name: ___	**DAY 20** 1. Mom Massage 2. Meals 3. Errands 4. Social Hour Name: ___	**DAY 21** 1. Mom Massage 2. Meals 3. Errands 4. Social Hour Name: ___
DAY 22 1. Mom Massage 2. Meals 3. Errands 4. Social Hour Name: ___	**DAY 23** 1. Mom Massage 2. Meals 3. Errands 4. Social Hour Name: ___	**DAY 24** 1. Mom Massage 2. Meals 3. Errands 4. Social Hour Name: ___	**DAY 25** 1. Mom Massage 2. Meals 3. Errands 4. Social Hour Name: ___	**DAY 26** 1. Mom Massage 2. Meals 3. Errands 4. Social Hour Name: ___	**DAY 27** 1. Mom Massage 2. Meals 3. Errands 4. Social Hour Name: ___	**DAY 28** 1. Mom Massage 2. Meals 3. Errands 4. Social Hour Name: ___
DAY 29 1. Mom Massage 2. Meals 3. Errands 4. Social Hour Name: ___	**DAY 30** 1. Mom Massage 2. Meals 3. Errands 4. Social Hour Name: ___	**DAY 31** 1. Mom Massage 2. Meals 3. Errands 4. Social Hour Name: ___	**DAY 32** 1. Postpartum Bath 2. Change Bed 3. Meals 4. Hold Baby	**DAY 33** 1. Mon Massage 2. Belly Bind 3. Meals 4. Social	**DAY 34** 1. Sleep 2. Mom Massage 3. Meals 4. Errands	**DAY 35** 1. Shower 2. Meals 3. Hold Baby 4. Social Hour
DAY 36 1. Postpartum Bath 2. Change Bed 3. Meals Name: ___	**DAY 37** 1. Herbal Teas 2. Meals 3. Nap 4. Social Time Name: ___	**DAY 38** 1. Hold Baby 2. Mom Massage 3. Chores Name: ___	**DAY 39** 1. Postpartum Bath 2. Change Bed 3. Meals 4. Hold Baby Name: ___	**DAY 40** 1. Herbal Teas 2. Meals 3. Nap 4. Social Time Name: ___	**DAY 41** 1. Mom Massage 2. Meals 3. Nap 4. Errands Name: ___	**DAY 42** 1. Postpartum Bath 2. Change Bed 3. Meals 4. Circle the House Name: ___

The calendar lists things a mother needs to help with postpartum recuperation, and who can assist her. The social hours can be shortened.

Acknowledgments

THANK YOU TO MY ANCESTORS AND THE GRANNY MIDWIVES, whose life's work has inspired me. I thank my parents, Yvonne D. and Thomas W. Monroe, for all that they poured into me: their love, values, and teaching me to give back to my community. To my beloved husband, Mikal H. Shabazz, whose consistent support has been a steady force in helping me complete this book. And to my exceptional children: Abdul Latif, Amenyonah Majeeda-Kenza, Moses Musa, Makeda Johari, Kamaria Aina, Isaiah Maun, Sharnissa Twana, and Nia Asibi—my constant cheerleaders, you each remind me why legacy matters. Thank you to my beautiful grandchildren for their belief in my work and to all my friends for your consistent encouragement.

I am profoundly grateful to Erykah Badu, a five-time GRAMMY award winner, for the honor of writing my foreword, and I extend a special thank-you to James Beard Award–winning author Michael W. Twitty for his support and advice in creating my book proposal, and to my friend and colleague Dr. Aviva Romm for her pivotal role in connecting me with my book agent. Deep appreciation to my daughter, Amenyonah Bossman, for the original creation of the Postpartum Care Calendar. Deep thanks to Sabreee's Gullah Art Gallery for the beautiful illustration on the cover.

I believe that every author and editor has a sacred relationship, and that has been true of my work with Colleen Martell, who was a wonderful guide, supporter, and partner through this entire writing process. Remember, you're never too far postpartum to follow the teachings and heal. Thank you also to my agents, Ericka Phillips and Stephanie Tade, whose guidance and expertise made this big project feel possible and doable. To my entire team at Balance, especially Renee Sedliar, who tirelessly shepherded me through many drafts: thank you.

Above all, I am most grateful to the Creator for the inspiration to write a book that helps new mothers and future generations of mothers be healthy during their postpartum period.

Notes

Introduction: How I Became "Queen Mother" of a Midwife Movement

1. Donna L. Hoyert, PhD, "Maternal Mortality Rates in the United States, 2021," *National Center for Health Statistics, Health E-Stats* (2023), https://dx.doi.org/10.15620/cdc:124678.

2. Johns Hopkins Medicine, "Four Common Pregnancy Complications," accessed June 3, 2025, https://www.hopkinsmedicine.org/health/conditions-and-diseases/staying-healthy-during-pregnancy/4-common-pregnancy-complications#:-:text=Most%20pregnancies%20progress%20without%20incident,the%20mother%20or%20the%20baby.

Chapter 1: Reviving the Lost Traditions of the African American Granny Midwife

1. Hanna Hill, "The History of Black Midwives in America," accessed June 3, 2025, https://www.hannahillphotography.com/blog-education/the-history-of-black-midwives.

2. Gertrude Jacinta Fraser, *African American Midwifery in the South: Dialogues of Birth, Race, and Memory* (Harvard University Press, 1998), 259.

3. Ibid.

4. Herbert C. Covey, *African American Slave Medicine: Herbal and Non-Herbal Treatments* (Lexington Books, 2008).

5. *Bringin' in Da Spirit*, directed by Rhonda L. Haynes (Alexander Street Press, 2003).

6. Wendy Bovard and Gladys Milton, *Why Not Me?: The Story of Gladys Milton, Midwife* (Book Publishing Company, 1993).

7. Onnie Lee Logan and Katherine Clark, *Motherwit: An Alabama Midwife's Story* (Plume, 1989).

8. Omar Shabazz, personal account to author, 2017.

9. Fraser, *African American Midwifery in the South*.

10. *Bringin' in Da Spirit*, directed by Haynes.

11. Sallie Ann Robinson, *Gullah Home Cooking the Daufuskie Way: Smokin' Joe Butter Beans, Ol' 'Fuskie Fried Crab Rice, Sticky-Bush Blackberry Dumpling, and Other Sea Island Favorites* (University of North Carolina Press, 2014).

12. Carol S. Johnston and Cindy A. Gaas, "Vinegar: Medicinal Uses and Antiglycemic Effect," *MedGenMed* 8(2) (2006): 61, https://pubmed.ncbi.nlm.nih.gov/16926800/.

13. Mikiya Kishi et al., "Enhancing Effect of Dietary Vinegar on the Intestinal Absorption of Calcium in Ovariectomized Rats," *Bioscience, Biotechnology, and Biochemistry* 63(5) (1999): 905–910, https://academic.oup.com/bbb/article-abstract/63/5/905/5 946568.

14. Sydney Shead, "'Granny' Midwife to Nurse-Midwife: The Decline of Southern Black Midwifery in the 20th Century," *Historical Perspectives: Santa Clara University Undergraduate Journal of History, Series II* 27(9) (2002), https://scholarcommons .scu.edu/historical-perspectives/vol27/iss1/9.

15. Laurie A. Wilkie, *The Archaeology of Mothering: An African-American Midwife's Tale* (Routledge, 2003).

16. *Bringin' in Da Spirit*, directed by Haynes.

17. (Monroe, S., 2018).p. 34

18. Marie Campbell, *Folks Do Get Born* (Rinehart & Company, 1946).

19. Wilkie, *The Archaeology of Mothering*.

Chapter 2: Sankofa: Stirring Up Healing Traditions

1. Maya Miller, "As Midwifery Evolves, This Mississippi Museum Is Preserving the History of Granny Midwives," WBHM, accessed March 23, 2023, https://wbhm.org /2023/as-midwifery-evolves-this-mississippi-museum-is-preserving-the-history-of -granny-midwives/.

2. *Bringin' in Da Spirit*, directed by Rhonda L. Haynes (Alexander Street Press, 2003).

3. Ibid.

4. American College of Obstetricians and Gynecologists, "Optimizing Postpartum Care," accessed June 3, 2025, https://www.acog.org/clinical/clinical-guidance/committee -opinion/articles/2018/05/optimizing-postpartum-care.

5. Niara Sudarkasa, *The Strength of Our Mothers: African & African American Women & Families: Essays and Speeches* (Africa World Press, 1997).

6. Reyus Mammadli, "Infection After Miscarriage: Signs and Symptoms," *Health Recovery*, accessed June 3, 2025, https://iytmed.com/infection-after-miscarriage-signs -and-symptoms/.

Chapter 3: Honored and Prayed Over

1. Robert H. Keefe, Carol Brownstein-Evans, and Rebecca Rouland Polmanteer, "'I Find Peace There': How Faith, Church, and Spirituality Help Mothers of Colour Cope with Postpartum Depression," *Mental Health, Religion & Culture* 19(7) (2016): 722–733, https://doi.org/10.1080/13674676.2016.1244663.

2. Ibid.

3. Mary-Powel Thomas et al., "Doula Services Within a Healthy Start Program: Increasing Access for an Underserved Population," *Maternal and Child Health Journal*, 21(1) (2017): 59–64, https://pubmed.ncbi.nlm.nih.gov/29198051/.

4. Dr. Oscar Serrallach, *The Postnatal Depletion Cure: A Complete Guide to Rebuilding*

Your Health and Reclaiming Your Energy for Mothers of Newborns, Toddlers, and Young Children (Grand Central Publishing, 2018).

5. Laurie A. Wilkie, *The Archaeology of Mothering: An African-American Midwife's Tale* (Routledge, 2003).

6. Doris Noel Ugarriza, "Social Support Unique to African American Mothers," *Journal of African American Studies* 10 (2006): 19–31, https://doi.org/10.1007/s12111-006-1006-3.

7. Wilkie, *The Archaeology of Mothering*.

8. Gertrude Jacinta Fraser, *African American Midwifery in the South: Dialogues of Birth, Race, and Memory* (Harvard University Press, 1998).

Chapter 4: Warmed

1. WikiDiff, "Heat vs. Warmth—What's the Difference?," https://wikidiff.com/heat/warmth.

2. Gerard A. Malanga, Ning Yan, and Jill Stark, "Mechanisms and Efficacy of Heat and Cold Therapies for Musculosketal Injury," *Post Graduate Medicine* 127, no. 1 (2025): 57–65, https://doi.org/10.1080/00325481.2015.992719.

3. Christine Kovach, "Do Warmed Blankets Change Pain, Agitation, Mood, or Analgesic Use Among Nursing Home Residents?," *Innovation in Aging* 3, no. 1 (2019): S623, https://doi.org/10.1093/geroni/igz038.2320.

4. "How to Get a Good Immune System: A Comprehensive Guide," Cymbiotika Health Hub, accessed February 12, 2025, https://cymbiotika.com/blogs/health-hub/how-to-get-a-good-immune-system-a-comprehensive-guide A.

5. Pamela Mason, "Thermotherapy and Cryotherapy," *The Pharmaceutical Journal*, June 17, 2014, https://pharmaceutical-journal.com/article/ld/thermotherapy-and-cryotherapy?form=MG0AV3.

6. Simone Maree Ormsby, "Hot and Cold Theory: Evidence in Nutrition," in *Hot and Cold Theory: The Path Towards Personalized Medicine*, edited by Maryam Yavari (Springer, 2022): 87–107.

7. April J. Bell et al., "'This Sickness Is Not Hospital Sickness'": A Qualitative Study of the Evil Eye as a Source of Neonatal Illness in Ghana," *Journal of Biosocial Science* 52, no. 2 (June 2019): 159–167, https://doi.org/10.1017/S0021932019000312.

8. Meghann Batten, Eleanor Stevenson, Deb Zimmerman, and Christine Isaacs, "Implementation of Hydrotherapy Protocol to Improve Postpartum Pain in Management," *Journal of Midwifery Women's Health* 62, no. 2 (March 2017): 210–214.

9. Shinta Wurdiana Rhomadona and Danita Primihastuti, "Combination of Herbal Steam Bath and Endorphin Massage to Increase Breast Milk Production," *Journal of Midwifery* 8, no. 1 (July 2023): 12–23, https://doi.org/10.25077/jom.8.1.72-23.2023A.

10. Molly C. Dougherty, "Southern Lay Midwives as Ritual Specialists," in Judith Hoch-Smith and Anita Spring (eds.), *Women in Ritual and Symbolic Roles* (Plenum Press, 1978), 151–164.

Chapter 5: Cleansed

1. James Ramos, "AB 1041: Wildlife: White Sage: Taking and Possession," Digital Democracy, accessed June 3, 2025, https://calmatters.digitaldemocracy.org/bills/ca_202320240ab1041.

2. WebMD Editorial Contributor, "How to Dry Up Your Breast Milk Supply," medically reviewed by Traci C. Johnson, MD, on April 23, 2025, WebMD, accessed June 3, 2025, https://www.webmd.com/baby/how-to-dry-up-your-breast-milk-supply.

3. Rebecca C. Thurston, PhD, et al., "Prospective Evaluation of Nighttime Hot Flashes During Pregnancy and Postpartum," *Fertility and Sterility* 100(6) (2013), https://www.sciencedirect.com/science/article/pii/S0015028213029671.

4. Cleveland Clinic, "Postpartum Night Sweats," last reviewed January 18, 2023, https://my.clevelandclinic.org/health/symptoms/24631-postpartum-night-sweats?form=MG0AV3&form=MG0AV3.

5. Junzhiwei Jiang et al., "Effects of Indoor Plants on CO_2 Concentration, Indoor Air Temperature and Relative Humidity in Office Buildings," *PLoS One* 9(7) (2024), https://pmc.ncbi.nlm.nih.gov/articles/PMC11253968/.

6. Jane Tarran, Fraser R. Torpy, and Margaret D. Burchett, "Use of Living Pot-Plants to Cleanse Indoor Air—Research Review," *Environmental Science* (2008), https://www.semanticscholar.org/paper/USE-OF-LIVING-POT-PLANTS-TO-CLEANSE-INDOOR-AIR-%E2%80%93-Tarran-Torpy/7a40ca80ecd03fe5701244b94c504620540e4543.

7. Jae-Won Yang et al., "Effects of Using Natural and Artificial Flowers in Flower Arrangement on Psychological and Physiological Relaxation," *Journal of People Plants Environment* 25(1) (2022): 39–48, https://doi.org/10.11628/ksppe.2022.25.1.39.

8. Shariful Islam et al., "A Study on the Human Health Benefits, Human Comfort Properties and Ecological Influences of Natural Sustainable Textile Fibers," *European Journal of Physiotherapy and Rehabilitation Studies* 1(1) (2020), https://oapub.org/hlt/index.php/EJPRS/article/view/47.

9. Antwon T. Chavis, MD, "Paternal Perinatal Depression in Modern-Day Fatherhood," *Pediatrics in Review* 43(10) (2022): 539–548, https://doi.org/10.1542/pir.2021-005488.

Chapter 6: Nourished

1. Helen Mendes, *The African Heritage Cookbook* (New York: The Macmillan Company, 1971).

2. Dr. Oscar Serrallach, *The Postnatal Depletion Cure: A Complete Guide to Rebuilding Your Health and Reclaiming Your Energy for Mothers of Newborns, Toddlers, and Young Children* (Grand Central Publishing, 2018).

3. Lisa Wartenberg, MFA, RD, LD, "How Much Iron Should You Be Getting Daily?," Healthline, medically reviewed by Katherine Marengo, LDN, RD, on December 9, 2019, accessed June 3, 2025, https://www.healthline.com/nutrition/how-much-iron-per-day#recommendations.

4. WebMD Editorial Contributor, "Hibiscus Tea: Is It Good for You?," medically reviewed by Zilpah Sheikh on November 16, 2023, WebMD, https://www.webmd.com/diet/hibiscus-tea-is-it-good-for-you.

5. S. A. Odunfa, "African Fermented Foods: From Art to Science," *MIRCEN Journal of Applied Microbiology and Biotechnology* 4 (1988): 259–273, https://link.springer.com/article/10.1007/bf01096132.

6. Charles M. A. P. Franz et al., "African Fermented Foods and Probiotics," *International Journal of Food Microbiology* 190 (2014): 84–96, https://www.sciencedirect.com/science/article/abs/pii/S0168160514004371.

7. Pallabi Banerjee and Imteyaz Qamar, "Chapter 6—Insights into the Technological and Nutritional Aspects of Lactic Milk Drinks: Buttermilk," *Advances in Dairy Microbial Products* (2022): 93–103, www.sciencedirect.com/science/article/abs/pii/B9780323857932000023.

8. Rakhi Chakraborty and Swarnendu Roy, "Exploration of the Diversity and Associated Health Benefits of Traditional Pickles from the Himalayan and Adjacent Hilly Regions of Indian Subcontinent," *Journal of Food Science and Technology* 55 (2018): 1599–1613, https://doi.org/10.1007/s13197-018-3080-7.

9. National Council on Aging, "Osteoporosis: The Risk Factors for Black Women," January 10, 2024, accessed June 3, 2025, https://www.ncoa.org/article/osteoporosis-the-risk-factors-for-black-women.

10. Jun Lv et al., "Consumption of Spicy Foods and Total and Cause Specific Mortality: Population Based Cohort Study," *BMJ* 351 (2015), https://www.bmj.com/content/351/bmj.h3942.short.

11. Grace Kuto, *Harambee! Stories and Recipes from the African Family Circle* (Best-Seller Books, 2008).

12. Vertamae Smart-Grosvenor, *Vibration Cooking: Or, The Travel Notes of a Geechee Girl* (University of Georgia Press, 2011).

13. David O. Kennedy, "B Vitamins and the Brain: Mechanisms, Dose and Efficacy — A Review," *Nutrients* 8(2) (2016): 68, https://www.mdpi.com/2072-6643/8/2/68?uid=662ec111s16.

14. Kyaien O. Conner, PhD, "Why Historical Trauma Is Critical to Understanding Black Mental Health," *Psychology Today*, October 1, 2020, https://www.psychologytoday.com/us/blog/achieving-health-equity/202010/why-historical-trauma-is-critical-understanding-black-mental.

Chapter 7: Hydrated and Healed

1. Droteea Teoibas-Serban et al., "Water Intake Meets the Water from Inside the Human Body—Physiological, Cultural, and Health Perspectives—Synthetic and Systematic Literature Review," *Balneo and PRM Research Journal* 12(3) (2021), https://bioclima.ro/Journal/index.php/BRJ/article/view/31.

2. Wikipedia, "African-American History," accessed June 3, 2025, https://en.wikipedia.org/w/index.php?title=African-American_history&oldid=1293688100.

3. Marc Williams, "African American Herbalism: A Blog Series," Chestnut School of Herbal Medicine, accessed June 3, 2025, https://chestnutherbs.com/african-american-herbalism-part-2/.

4. Yasuyuki Nemoto, "Messages from Water and 'New Science of Water,'" *Journal of International Society of Life Information Science* 33(1) (2015): 105, https://www.jstage.jst.go.jp/article/islis/33/1/33_KJ00009847732/_article.

5. Mahsa Maghalian et al., "The Effects of Warm Perineal Compress on Perineal Trauma and Postpartum Pain: A Systematic Review with Meta-Analysis and Trial Sequential Analysis," *Archives of Gynecology and Obstetrics*, 309(3) (2024): 843–869, https://doi.org/10.1007/s00404-023-07195-2.

6. Rena Goldman, "What Is Comfrey?," medically reviewed by Angelica Balingit, MD, updated on September 26, 2024, Healthline, accessed June 3, 2025, https://www.healthline.com/health/what-is-comfrey.

7. Jane Henderson, Fiona Alderdice, and Maggie Redshaw, "Factors Associated with Maternal Postpartum Fatigue: An Observational Study," *BMJ Open* 9 (2019), https://bmjopen.bmj.com/content/9/7/e025927.abstract.

8. Colleen de Bellefonds, "Postpartum Sweating," What to Expect, medically reviewed by James Greenberg, MD, on January 14, 2022, accessed June 3, 2025, https://www.whattoexpect.com/first-year/postpartum-health-and-care/postpartum-sweating/.

Chapter 8: Rested

1. John DeLucchi, PT, SCS, "Sleep: The Secret Ingredient of Injury Recovery," OrthoCarolina, accessed June 3, 2025, https://www.orthocarolina.com/media/sleep-the-secret-ingredient-of-injury-recovery.

2. Erika Schwartz and Jill Ketner Villa, "Navigating the Postpartum Period: Hormonal Changes and Essential Care for Women," in *Postpartum Period for Mother and Newborn* [Working Title] (IntechOpen, 2025).

3. Jennifer L. Weinberg, MD, MPH, MBE, "The Science of Sleep: Functional Medicine for Restorative Sleep," Rupa Health, accessed June 3, 2025, https://www.rupahealth.com/post/the-science-of-sleep-functional-medicine-for-restorative-sleep.

4. Stacy Liberatore, "The Science Behind the 'Golden Hour' After Birth: Experts Reveal Why the First 60 Minutes of Skin-to-Skin Contact Is Vital for Both the Mother and Newborn," *Daily Mail*, March 15, 2023, https://www.dailymail.co.uk/sciencetech/article-11863467/Experts-reveal-60-minutes-skin-skin-contact-vital-mother-newborn.html.

5. Therese Doan, PhD, et al., "Nighttime Breastfeeding Behavior Is Associated with More Nocturnal Sleep Among First-Time Mothers at One Month Postpartum," *Journal of Clinical Sleep Medicine* 10(3) (2014), https://jcsm.aasm.org/doi/pdf/10.5664/jcsm.3538.

6. Mark D. Mackenzie et al., "Adolescent Perspectives of Bedtime Social Media Use: A Qualitative Systematic Review and Thematic Synthesis," *Sleep Medicine Reviews* 63 (2022), https://doi.org/10.1016/j.smrv.2022.101626.

7. Jeffrey Gottfried, "Americans' Social Media Use," Pew Research Center, January 31, 2014, https://www.pewresearch.org/internet/2024/01/31/americans-social-media-use/.

8. Claire McCarthy, MD, "Room Sharing with Your Baby May Help Prevent SIDS, but It Means Everyone Gets Less Sleep," *Harvard Health Publishing*, August 16, 2020, https://www.health.harvard.edu/blog/room-sharing-with-your-baby-may-help-prevent-sids-but-it-means-everyone-gets-less-sleep-201706062525#:-:text=According%20to%20the%20American%20Academy,Infant%20Death%20Syndrome%2C%20or%20SIDS.

9. Diane Wiessinger et al., "The Safe Sleep Seven," in *Sweet Sleep: Nighttime and Naptime Strategies for the Breastfeeding Family* (Ballantine Books, 2014).

10. La Leche League International, "The Safe Sleep Seven," November 28, 2018, https://llli.org/news/the-safe-sleep-seven/.

Chapter 9: Loved

1. National Institutes of Health, "Brain Changes Observed During Pregnancy," October 1, 2024, https://www.nih.gov/news-events/nih-research-matters/brain-changes-observed-during-pregnancy.

2. John T. Chissell, *Pyramids of Power! An Ancient African Centered Approach to Optimal Health* (Positive Perceptions Publications, 1993).

3. Joni Sweet, "Breastfeeding and Breast Cancer: Does Breastfeeding Lower Breast Cancer Risk," Breast Cancer Research Foundation, n.d., https://www.bcrf.org/about-breast-cancer/breastfeeding-breast-cancer-risk/; Serena Crawford, "How Breast Feeding Lowers Mothers' Risk of Developing Type 2 Diabetes," Yale School of Medicine, July 18, 2023, https://medicine.yale.edu/news-article/how-breastfeeding-lowers-the-risk-of-developing-type-2-diabetes/; Biology Insights, "Anemia and Breastfeeding: How It Affects Mothers and Babies," April 29, 2025, https://biologyinsights.com/anemia-and-breastfeeding-how-it-affects-mothers-and-babies/.

4. Latif M. Bossman, *Prison Fathers: Parenting Behind Bars* (CreateSpace Independent Publishing Platform, 2018).

5. Kandace Redd, "Study: Black Dads More Involved in Activities with Their Children Than Other Groups," ABC10, January 17, 2024, https://www.abc10.com/article/news/community/race-and-culture/black-dads-more-involved-in-childrens-lives-than-other-groups/103-df371add-144c-40e3-bb3c-986377347fa1.

6. Stephanie Watson, "Forming a Bond with Your Baby—Why It Isn't Always Immediate," medically reviewed by Dan Brennan, MD, on August 8, 2024, WebMD, accessed June 3, 2025, https://www.webmd.com/parenting/baby/forming-a-bond-with-your-baby-why-it-isnt-always-immediate.

7. Andrea O'Reilly, *Toni Morrison and Motherhood: A Politics of the Heart* (State University of New York Press, 2004).

Chapter 10: Recipes for Healing, Strength, and Beauty

1. Vertamae Smart-Grosvenor, *Vibration Cooking: Or, The Travel Notes of a Geechee Girl* (University of Georgia Press, 2011).

2. Judith Carney, *Black Rice: The African Origins of Rice Cultivation in the Americas* (Harvard University Press, 2001), 32; Michael W. Twitty, *The Cooking Gene: A Journey Through African American Culinary History in the Old South* (HarperCollins, 2017), 4.

3. D. G. Coursey, "The Origins and Domestication of Yams in Africa," in B. Swartz and R. Dumett (eds.), *West African Culture Dynamics: Archaeological and Historical Perspectives* (Walter de Gruyter, 1980), 67–90, https://doi.org/10.1515/9783110800685.67.

4. Ariana Saraiva et al., "Coconut Sugar: Chemical Analysis and Nutritional Profile; Health Impacts; Safety and Quality Control; Food Industry Applications," *International Journal of Environmental Research and Public Health* 20(4) (2023): 3671, https://www.mdpi.com/1660-4601/20/4/3671.

5. Joe Schwarcz, PhD, "Chicken Soup's Label as 'Jewish Penicillin' Is More Whimsy Than Fact," McGill University Office of Science and Society, January 26, 2024, https://www.mcgill.ca/oss/article/health-and-nutrition-history/chicken-soups-label-jewish-penicillin-more-whimsy-fact.

6. Joe Leech, MS, "11 Proven Benefits of Garlic," medically reviewed by Jared Meacham, PhD, Healthline, accessed June 3, 2025, https://www.healthline.com/nutrition/11-proven-health-benefits-of-garlic#boosts-immune-system.

7. Stephanie Butler, "Hoppin' John: A New Year's Tradition," History Channel, December 28, 2012, https://www.history.com/articles/hoppin-john-a-new-years-tradition.

8. Dr. Sruthi M., "Are Turnip Greens Healthy? 10 Health Benefits," MedicineNet, n.d., https://www.medicinenet.com/are_turnip_greens_healthy/article.htm.

9. Sallie Ann Robinson, *Gullah Home Cooking the Daufuskie Way: Smokin' Joe Butter Beans, Ol' 'Fuskie Fried Crab Rice, Sticky-Bush Blackberry Dumpling, and Other Sea Island Favorites* (University of North Carolina Press, 2014).

10. Sarah Wassberg Johnson, "Meatless Monday: Easy Rice Pudding," *The Food Historian*, April 26, 2021, https://www.thefoodhistorian.com/blog/meatless-monday-easy-rice-pudding.

11. Peggy Aoki, "The History of Coconut Cake Is a Legacy of Black Cooking," Tasting Table, May 6, 2024, https://www.tastingtable.com/1576070/history-of-coconut-cake.

Chapter 11: Traditions and Rituals

1. Alameda Health System, "In Honor of Black History Month We Spotlight the Granny Midwives and Their Legacy," accessed June 3, 2025, https://www.alameda-healthsystem.org/honoring-the-granny-midwives-and-their-legacy/.

2. Michael Twitty, *The Cooking Gene: A Journey Through African American Culinary History in the Old South* (HarperCollins, 2017).

3. Gladys Milton, *Beyond the Storm: An Extraordinary Journey* (Boaz Fulwylie Press, 1997).

4. Laurie A. Wilkie, *The Archaeology of Mothering: An African-American Midwife's Tale* (Routledge, 2003).

5. Linda Janet Holmes, *Safe in a Midwife's Hands: Birthing Traditions from Africa to the American South* (The Ohio State University Press, 2023).

6. Patrick Macleod, "'Calming Watercolors': Using Mindful Art in Treatment of Mood Disorders," *Expressive Therapies Capstone Theses* (2020), 256, https://digitalcommons.lesley.edu/expressive_theses/256/.

7. For step-by-step instructions on how to properly complete postpartum belly binding, sign up for SMC Full Circle Doula's African American Postpartum Belly

Binding Webinar, https://smcdoulas.com/african-american-postpartum-belly-binding-webinar/.

8. Shafia Monroe, "African American Postpartum Belly Binding," accessed June 3, 2025, https://shafiamonroe.com/african-american-postpartum-belly-binding/.

9. Holmes, *Safe in a Midwife's Hands*.

Chapter 12: Improving Pregnancy Outcomes for Black Women

1. Areesha Lodhi, "Why Does the US Have Such a High Maternal Mortality Rate?," *Aljazeera*, August 17, 2024, https://www.aljazeera.com/news/2024/8/17/why-does-the-us-have-such-a-high-maternal-mortality-rate.

2. CDC, "Pregnancy-Related Deaths: Data from Maternal Mortality Review Committees in 38 U.S. States, 2020," May 28, 2024, https://www.cdc.gov/maternal-mortality/php/data-research/index.html.

3. Amnesty International, "Amnesty International Report 2022/23: The State of the World's Human Rights," n.d., https://www.amnesty.org/en/wp-content/uploads/2023/03/WEBPOL1056702023ENGLISH.pdf.

4. CommonSense Childbirth, "The JJ Way—a Patient-Centered Model of Care," n.d., https://commonsensechildbirth.org/the-jj-way/.

5. Eliza Barclay, "How Soul Food Can Be Good for Your Health," NPR, November 10, 2011, https://www.publicradiotulsa.org/2011-11-10/how-african-americans-can-get-healthy-with-big-helpings-of-soul-food.

6. Rekiku Fikre et al., "Effectiveness of Midwifery-Led Care on Pregnancy Outcomes in Low- and Middle-Income Countries: A Systematic Review and Meta-Analysis," *BMC Pregnancy and Childbirth* 23 (2023), https://bmcpregnancychildbirth.biomedcentral.com/articles/10.1186/s12884-023-05664-9.

7. Kathleen Knocke et al., "Doula Care and Maternal Health: An Evidence Review," ASPE Office of Health Policy, December 13, 2022, https://aspe.hhs.gov/reports/doula-care.

8. Annalies Winny and Rachel Bervell, MD, "How Can We Solve the Black Maternal Health Crisis?," Johns Hopkins Bloomberg School of Public Health, May 12, 2023, https://publichealth.jhu.edu/2023/solving-the-black-maternal-health-crisis.

9. Omoniyi Adebisi and Gregory Strayhorn, "Anemia in Pregnancy and Race in the United States: Blacks at Risk," *Family Medicine* 37(9) (2005): 655–662, https://pubmed.ncbi.nlm.nih.gov/16193419/.

10. Irogue Igbinosa et al., "Racial and Ethnic Disparities in Anemia and Severe Maternal Morbidity," *Obstretrics and Gynecology* 142(4) (2023): 845–854, https://pubmed.ncbi.nlm.nih.gov/37678935/.

11. Eghosa Ekhator, Servel Miller, and Etinosa Igbinosa, *Implementing the Sustainable Development Goals in Nigeria: Barriers, Prospects and Strategies* (Routledge, 2021).

12. Enav Yefet et al., "Good Glycemic Control of Gestational Diabetes Mellitus Is Associated with the Attenuation of Future Maternal Cardiovascular Risk: A Retrospective Cohort Study," *Cardiovascular Diabetology* 18(1) (2019): 75, https://pubmed.ncbi.nlm.nih.gov/31167664/.

INDEX

meat
  animal-derived iron, 133–134
  beef, 216–217, 223–224, 228
  chicken, 30–31, 159, 211–212, 214–215,
    220–221, 226, 229–230
  eggs, 31, 210–211
  fish and shellfish, 213, 217–219,
    224–225, 230–231
  goat, 222–223
  lamb, 227
medical negligence, 184
melanin, 80–81
Mendes, Helen, 127
menopause, 95–96
menstrual pads, 116–117
menstruation, 116–117, 160–161
Mexican traditions, 14
midwifery. *See also* African American
    Granny Midwife
  African American definition of
    midwife, 18–19
  Mississippi Black midwives, 9, 63
  permits, regulation, and, 33–34
  reviving lost traditions of African
    American Granny Midwife,
    13–37
  training, 13–14, 28
  Tuskegee School of
    Nurse-Midwifery and, 34
Milton, Gladys, 23–24, 245
mindset, for positive pregnancy and
    birth, 265–267
mint tea, 27
miscarriage, 65
Mississippi Black midwives, 9, 63
Moon, Layla, 264
Morrison, Toni, 197

motherhood
  asking and receiving questions
    about, 79–80
  as blessing, 192–196
  celebrating power of, 65–66, 193–196
  community mothering and, 26–27
  fusing over the mother, 57–58
  honoring, 71–72, 75–80, 87, 274–275
  "losing yourself" to, 194–195
  loving, 192–196
  mothering the mother and, 50–52
  negative associations with, 46–48,
    192–194
  prayer for protection of mother
    and, 259
  racism and, 192–193, 260–261
  as rite of passage, 51–52, 85
  stay-at-home mothers and, 47
  transitioning to, 13–14
  under Western medical model, 45–49
Motherwit
  African American Granny Midwife
    and, 19–23
  Black women and, 19–23, 75–80
  dismissal of, 22–23
  honoring yourself and, 75–76,
    78–80, 274–275
  inner knowing and, 20–23
  postpartum care and, 19–23
Muhammad, Elijah, 127
muscle injuries, 157
myrrh, 113

naming baby, 255–256
National Maternity and Infancy
    Protection Act (1921)
    (Sheppard-Towner Act), 33

recipes (*cont.*)
    for lying-in period, 209–220
    for meals, 220–232
    Postpartum Iron Healing Tea
      Recipe, 138
    soup and stew, 207–209, 211–231
    for sweets and desserts, 235–239
    for tea, 233–235
reclaiming culture and tradition, 7–8,
    21, 36–37, 39–41, 60
red clover, 136, 154, 161, 163
red raspberry leaf, 137, 138, 154
regulation, of midwifery, 33–34
relaxation, 29. *See also* rest
    de-stressing practices and,
      266–267
    Relaxing Tea, 233–234
    tea for, 121–122, 154, 176, 233–234
    warmth and, 94, 248
relaxin, 49
religion, 110–111
respect
    for African American Granny
      Midwife, 5, 25–26
    prayer, honor, and, 63
rest
    African American ancestral
      healing traditions for, 165–178
    baths for, 176, 187
    difference between rest and sleep,
      169–172
    fatigue, tiredness, and, 168–169
    healing and, 64
    how to, 170–171
    immediately postpartum, 171–172
    importance of, 165–167
    internet, cell phones, and, 174–175

    during lying-in period, 167–168, 171
    massage and, 176
    postpartum care and, 17–18, 35
    practicing, 50–51
    prayer for, 165
    rituals for, 248
    self-care and, 71
    sleep and, 29, 169–172
    tips for creating ease with, 61
Rhimes, Shonda, 264
rice
    Rice Porridge, 27–28, 209–210
    Rice Pudding, 236
rite of passage
    cooking as, 144
    motherhood as, 51–52, 85
    postpartum period as, 51–52, 85
rituals
    African American ancestral
      healing traditions and, 241–257
    for any time, 58
    baby-naming ceremony and,
      255–256
    bathing, 103–104, 246–247
    beautifying, 81, 244–245
    belly wrapping, 241–242, 247,
      249–251
    call-and-response prayer and,
      83–84
    circle the house, 248–249
    cleanliness and, 243–244
    cleansing, 110–113, 123
    communal care and, 245
    elders and, 241–243
    environment for, 244
    foundation of African American
      postpartum, 243–245

shrinking uterus (involution), 99,
161
SisterSong Women of Color
Reproductive Justice Collective,
56–57
sitz bath, 158, 176
skin-to-skin contact, 98, 171, 256
slavery
African American history and, 4, 5,
18, 77, 81–82, 165–166
babies and, 77
post-traumatic slave syndrome
and, 77
Transatlantic Slave Trade and, 18
sleep
during any time of day, 176–177
for babies, 177–178
co-sleeping and bed-sharing, 178
difference between rest and,
169–172
environment for, 173–174
during hospital stay, 172–173
how to get good sleep, 172–178
importance of, 166–167
Mama Shafia's Twelve Tips for
Good Sleep, 176–177
relaxation and, 29
rest and, 29, 169–172
Safe Sleep Seven guidelines, 178
sleepy-time tea, 154
Smart-Grosvenor, Vertamae, 202
Smith, Claudine Curry, 45
smoking rituals, 112–113
snacks, 122, 140–141
social media, 146
social support, 50–52. *See also*
community mothering model

community support and, 58–59,
60–62, 245
prayer and, 69–70
soup and stew, 126
as *the* African American
postpartum food, 207–208
Beef and Turnip Stew, 228
Beef Stew, 223–224
Black-Eyed Pea, Spinach, and Fish
Soup, 217–218
bone broth, 30
broth, 30, 153–156
Browned Goat Stew, 222–223
chicken, 30–31, 159
Chicken Vegetable Soup, 211–212
Coconut Shrimp Soup, 213
Curried Chicken, Mixed Greens,
and Coconut Soup, 214–215
Green Bean and Brown Chicken
Stew, 226
Groundnut Soup, 212
Hoppin' John Shrimp Stew,
224–225
Lamb, Kale, Potato Stew, 227
Liver and Fig Stew, 220–221
Oxtail Red Bean Soup, 219–220
Palm Oil Soup, 228–229
Peanut Butter Soup, 212
Pepper and Hominy Grit Stew,
225–226
recipes, 207–209, 211–231
Seafood Gumbo, 230–231
Spinach Garlic Stew with
Chicken, 214
Succotash Stew, 221–222
Sweet Potato, Ginger, Chicken
Soup, 229–230